BPD Voices Project Vol. 1

A collection of experiences from those who live with Borderline Personality Disorder

*BPD Pieces of me Community
Introduction by:
Melanie Carrillo*

Thank you for purchasing this book.

All proceeds benefit BPD Pieces of Me, which is a non-profit organization dedicated to providing education and support for individuals, families, friends, and providers living with borderline personality disorder.

Our vision is for all person's with borderline personality disorder to have online access and support to mental health and wellness programs.

BPD Voices Project
Copyright © 2016 by Melanie Carrillo
Cover Art Copyright © 2016 by Hayley Figiel
Second Edition Back and White
ISBN: 978-1533243249
ISBN: 1533243247
Requests for information should be sent to:
BPDPiecesofMe@gmail.com

All rights reserved. No part of this publication may be reproduced, distributed, or transmitted in any form or by any means, including photocopying, recording, or other electronic or mechanical methods, without the prior written permission of the publisher, except in the case of brief quotations embodied in critical reviews and certain other noncommercial uses permitted by copyright law. For permission requests, write to the publisher, addressed "Attention: Permissions Coordinator," to BPDPiecesofMe@gmail.com.

All stories, poems, quotes, and art work, have been printed with written permission of the author or artist. Each author or artist is the sole copy write owner and retains all rights to their printed work.

This book is not intended as a substitute for the medical advice of physicians. The reader should regularly consult a physician in matters relating to his/her health and particularly with respect to any symptoms that may require diagnosis or medical attention.

Although the editors and publisher have made every effort to ensure that the information in this book was correct at press time, the editors and publisher do not assume and hereby disclaim any liability to any party for any loss, damage, or disruption caused by errors or omissions, whether such errors or omissions result from negligence, accident, or any other cause.

Submissions have been edited for clarity and grammar.

This book is dedicated to all who shared their experience of Borderline Personality Disorder with the project, and to all those who fight daily to eliminate the stigma surrounding this disorder.

Contents:

Introduction

I: Daily Living	1-60
II: Relationships	61-112
III. Suicide/Self Harm	113-156
IV: Effects of Abuse	157-206
V: Moments of Change	207-232
VI: Recovery	233-275
Index of Authors	276-279

Voices Project: Where's Your Voice?

I remember when I was first diagnosed with BPD. It was 2002. I was 26. A new mother living in rural New Hampshire. My family was 3,000 miles away on the whole other coast of the country. I felt isolated and alone. Spiraling deeper and deeper into the pit that is mental illness, I struggled. My family struggled. I was in and out of the hospital. Bi-polar? Postpartum psychosis?

No, Borderline Personality Disorder.

We all assumed the worse; I wouldn't make it thought the year. But I did, and I wanted to get better!

Back then my Internet still ran through a modem. Late at night I could get a decent connection but there wasn't much I could find about people experiencing BPD. Well I lie, I found a lot of information about how we were incurable monsters that should be avoided and or destroyed.

I was not that person! I wanted help! I wanted healing!

But today, things are different. The Internet provides a place of refuge and encouragement, and many have used the support to become well!

I discovered that there were many faces of BPD. The face of those who suffer. The face of those who live with those who suffer. The face of those who are friends with those who suffer.

The catalyst for change in the way BPD is perceived by others was many refused to be silent! They refused to be told what their illness should look like. Refused to believe there was no cure.

But many are still struggling to find their voice.

So I started a project titled the "BPD Voices Project" to give everyone a place to have a voice in the darkness. To give a voice to those who want to help in the fight against stigma and misunderstanding that surrounds BPD.

With the only requirement to be truthful, we asked for people to submit a short paragraph that speaks honestly about their experience with BPD.

Our first submission was anonymous:

Living with BPD is difficult. Not only is it one of the most stigmatized disorders, but not many people truly understand it. I'm going into clinical psychology, and I've discovered a sad truth; the majority of clinicians refuse to work with borderlines or they call them "tiring," "difficult," etc. I don't mean to be this way. I either feel nothing or everything at once, no in-between. A friend or significant other can do one thing and I automatically think they're bad. When I care about someone or something, I put all of my energy into it. I've used this for good, such as with school. I became obsessed with psychology when I was 16 years-old and as a result of that I have graduated two years early and am starting my doctorate in the fall. However, that passion also brings me the most pain. I know I will make a good clinician because I am so intuitive; I can figure out the source of almost any problem. I'm what they call a "high functioning borderline," which ironically makes it worse because people don't think anything is wrong. I will be fine one minute and then if something triggers me, I will be on the floor crying my eyes out. I know why I'm this way; my father was emotionally abusive and that's why I seek validation. I am proud of how far I've come, but I'm afraid I will always live with the fear of abandonment. It's so hard to be in a relationship because I end up projecting my fears onto them and push them away. I just need someone who understands. Until then, I will live with this pain and use my understanding of the disorder to help the millions of individuals living with it. – Anonymous

BPD recovery begins when voices are not only heard, but validated.

The project is meant to give us a place to speak our voice, tell our stories our way, not in the way professionals tell us we should. It gives us a platform to come together as a community to fight stigma and misunderstanding by letting people into our inner world to see the battles we face every day. A way to let them know the battles we have won.

The stories aren't often pretty, but they are as raw and true as the disorder itself.

In my humble opinion the project has been a big success and I look forward to many more voices being heard through this book. We have received submissions from around the world and one thing becomes apparent in our stories: we are not alone.

I hope this is a project that will go on for many years so that all may have a voice to heal.

Melanie Carrillo
Founder and President of BPD Pieces of Me

I.

Daily Living

Derailed

Broken and Shattered, Black and Blue
Words like daggers, Pierced flesh through and through
Silent unspoken fears from the past
The demons hold tightly, my minds bought to crash
Bust into the darkness, with head held up high
Keep searching for light rays, there's no need to cry
Crazy mayhem, wicked thoughts
Hands perspire, gut's in knots
Thoughts like a whirlwind, all twisted and torn
Have things been this fucked up, since the day I was born
Eyes heavy like big blocks of stone, I lay there agonizing inside my mind alone
My thoughts seem clearer in the darkness of night
Living inside my head all the time is a terrible fight
Pain is too large, It's so hard to sleep
Holding onto the memories, I don't want to keep
Where did they come from, why haven't they gone
My mind's getting tired of this repetitive song
Can't move forward, when I keep looking back
Live becomes more difficult, when you're stuck on this track
Release all this chaos from inside my brain
For I am the conductor of this crazy, fucked up train

Jennifer George
USA

Living with BPD is difficult. Not only is it one of the most stigmatized disorders, but not many people truly understand it. I'm going into clinical psychology, and I've discovered a sad truth; the majority of clinicians refuse to work with borderlines or they call them "tiring," "difficult," etc. I don't mean to be this way.

I either feel nothing or everything at once, no in-between. A friend or significant other can do one thing and I automatically think they're bad. When I care about someone or something, I put all of my energy into it. I've used this for good, such as with school. I became obsessed with psychology when I was 16 years-old and as a result of that I have graduated two years early and am starting my doctorate in the fall. However, that passion also brings me the most pain. I know I will make a good clinician because I am so intuitive; I can figure out the source of almost any problem.

I'm what they call a "high functioning borderline," which ironically makes it worse because people don't think anything is wrong. I will be fine one minute and then if something triggers me, I will be on the floor crying my eyes out. I know why I'm this way; my father was emotionally abusive and that's why I seek validation.

I am proud of how far I've come, but I'm afraid I will always live with the fear of abandonment. It's so hard to be in a relationship because I end up projecting my fears onto them and push them away. I just need someone who understands. Until then, I will live with this pain and use my understanding of the disorder to help the millions of individuals living with it.

Anonymous

I sit staring at myself in the mirror with this expression on my face as if I do not recognize the blob in front of me. I see a woman looking back at me that is not myself. Her vacant expression chills my soul. Her dark brown eyes scan over my empty soul and I cannot help but understand why.

She is I.

My numb, vacant soul desires for a taste of feeling that never comes. It is I that looks to the woman in the mirror for guidance. The guidance will never come. It is I that never commits and deep down I know the truth is a liar. I'm a work in progress. I'm a total disconnected masterpiece who wishes to feel.

Tiffany Rayborn
USA

To tell me I've made a mistake is to tell me I AM a mistake."

Jennifer Purvis
USA

I'm tired of being sad,
I'm tired of being mad.
I'm tired of feeling lonely,
And I'm tired of being isolated.

Yet I'm tired of being around people,
I'm tired of all these masks I wear.
I'm tired of daily life tasks being so much effort,
To the point I'm overwhelmed and wish I were dying.
I'm tired of crying and being a mess.
I'm sick of all the stress.
Why do I find every little thing so hard?
Sometimes i want to die, but I'm too scared.
It feels like I'm stuck here.
I'm sick of not knowing who I am, not liking what I see when I look in the mirror.
I'm sick of my financial status.
I'm sick of having no friends and feeling like I have no one.
I'm sick of feeling tired, and I'm tired of feeling sick.
I hate leaving my house.
I hate the way that I am.
I hate that I over think every little thing.
I hate that living is taking its toll on me.
I hate the fact that I was going to do an art work for this project and I couldn't.
I hate that my life is like this, and that it wont go away.
I just want to go away.
I'm sick of being judged,
I'm sick of trying to fit in.
I'm sick of being overwhelmed.
I'm sick of screaming.
I hate my life.
I hate feeling every emotion so intensely,
And I hate feeling absolutely nothing.
I hate that these moods fluctuate so fast,
Its the story of my life's past.
I've never known a different me.
But I don't know if this is me...
I'm tired of feeling abandoned and left out.

My life is such a contradiction.
My mind is a constant rollercoaster.
I just wish that it will all end.
No amount of words can describe how much
pain this all is, I don't even know if this is a
start...

Carly Simpson
New South Wales

Grey Matter

I'm no longer the person I was of years ago, I'm just the shell of what used to be. Broken, shattered pieces of a leader, a co-worker, of someone who people turned to for direction, for answers, for support. A girl who had dreams of making something, anything, better of her life.

I sit here today, with no direction, no real reason to wake some mornings. I am my own boss, the owner and employee of a creative and chaotic mind that is just screaming and begging for the wheels & cogs to a line. Some days it's too much, while other's it's not enough.

I need no judgment or ridicule, as I am more than capable of establishing elaborate criticisms in my own mind. Exploding emotions like red hot fireworks, creating problems when none exist, intensifying situations requiring stitches not just a band aid.

I am my worst enemy, the monster under the bed, the dark figure lurking in the shadows. I am my best friend, the voice of encouragement, the cheering section of life. I am my worst enemy, the terrorizing screams that discourages the cheering section to thrive, that suffocates any attempt at realizing my full potential.

I am either happy or sad, good or evil, I am the grey matter which floats through the atmosphere; struggling to find a way to dissipate, to break through into the brightness, the warming rays of sunshine, the melodic sounds of laughter amongst friends & loved ones.

I am a burden on my own destiny, as well as the key holder of my future. To be at odds with one's emotional existence, fighting for and against the rationality of words & actions, can create a bond that can't be broken or a platform for leaping head first into the thick muck of selfishness, and despair, anger, and frustration.

I am my own best and worst...

Jennifer George
USA

My armours dented
My shield is cracked
Still inside my heart beats
My lungs draw breath

The fires burn inside my chest
The lightning crackles through my eyes
An icy touch still chills my bones
My blood boils inside my veins

A forced smile; through gritted teeth
A mask to wear for all to see
I try my best to see the sun
But all I see is clouds

Rob Hernfield
Australia

Silent screams and silent tears
Lots of worries lots of fears

I don't want you to walk an inch in my shoes
That's a journey that no one should choose
My feet are aching my minds a mess
It's my road to walk down but it's hard to rest,

So when sometimes I ignore you in the street
And I just stare down at my feet.
Remember it's not that I don't care
It's just I have a mind that doesn't play fair.

Kirsty McCarthy
Wales

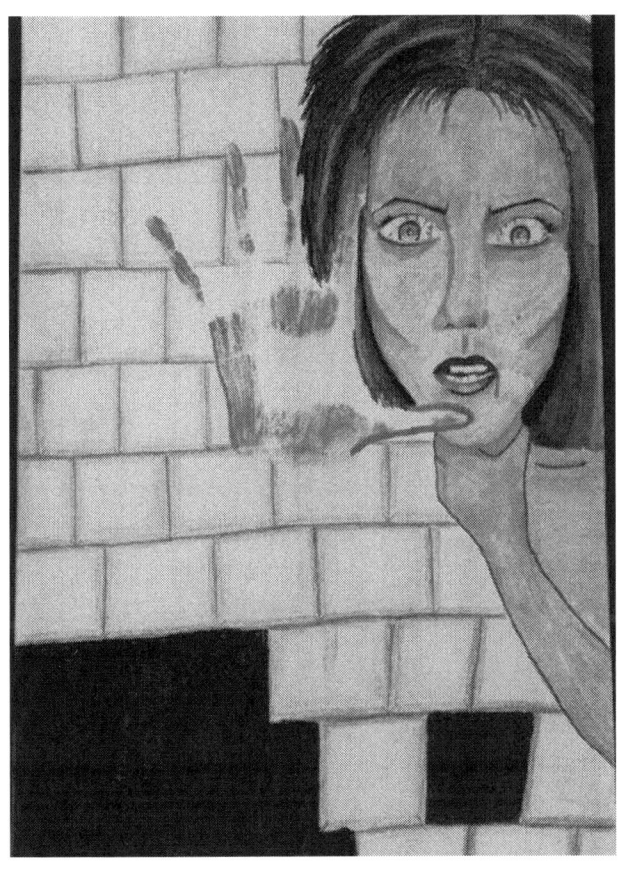

Pissed personality disorder

Mal Hultgren
Sweeden

Fighting an inner battle is the hardest thing to explain to anyone. How do you explain to someone about the demons who hold you hostage, that torture you, when they aren't real? They are real to me when I force myself to get out of bed, smile and say fine thank you when it's the last thing I feel like doing and I'm far from fine.

These demons are real when I feel my soul is broken, every chasing thought painful. So real when I feel nothing but despair, can't see myself in a happy future, the numbness takes over. When I try so hard to be positive, but find myself lost.

How many times and many ways I've seeked the answers, tried to get help...no pills could fix me (temporary help, relief but no cure)? How do I explain things I don't understand? When for no particular reason I get anxiety, become scared, feel lonely, get mad, upset want to shout and force people away from me? When I want to be by myself, or desperately need someone to hold me?

The deep infliction, wounds inside. From sad to glad, feeling overly excited, like you're on some natural high. Going from smelling the flowers, dancing in the rain, kissing rainbows, laughing like its the most beautiful thing, feeling in love to broken, exhausted, numb, empty, useless, not worthy.

Sometimes something little can be the trigger, other times nothing. This is my daily battle, for weeks or days or only hours demons I have to face... this be but a fraction of my reality. How would you explain them?

Freeda Du Plessis
South Africa

What if?

Hope disappears, sucked into the depths of the sewage that runs deep beneath our feet,
Where the rats carry the hidden diseases that infect my mind,
The darkness chokes me as I struggle for air,
But the secrets clench their bony fists tight around my neck,
The weight of shame resting on my hollow chest where once my heart beat strong,
It's now damaged from the rusty nails of broken promises, betrayal and evil words, that pierce deep into my weakened muscle,
I take the responsibility of turning these internal wounds into ugly scars upon my skin: where eyes look down with disappointment and disgust as I express my pain I have within.
Am I crazy? Am I insane? Am I deranged?
They fill my body with medications, these chemicals they say are for my own good, they pile them on I take them, but do they poison me, steal my identity, I do not know.
They place their labels upon my head, lock me up, and use their textbooks to manage me, control me, and then forget me.
Am I unfixable? Is that what they're trying to say?
Anger engulfs my mind, body and soul like a stormy wave takes a lonely shell on a deserted beach,
Swallowed by the surf, and drowned by the current.
My eyes, red and sore, from my salty tears that race down my pale skin like their trying to escape me too,
I am alone.
The voices in my head tell me to let go. What if I do? Even just for a second, a small moment in time? Would they notice? Would they care?
I dream of a life that's so peaceful, even the most fragile of beasts can survive there,

As beautiful as the delicate butterfly, recently emerged from its cocoon ready to spread its wings for the first time...
But dreams turn into nightmares, and this once magical place becomes dark and dangerous, where around every corner there's a new monster trying to knock you down.
I am afraid.
Scared like a small mouse in the middle of a herd of angry elephants,
Overwhelmed by a world of hate and rejection...
What if this is all there is for me?
What if this is my end?

Leanne Quinney
UK

Can I speak about myself?

I'm Amy wood, since being young I have always been "different"… I always longed for a Dad mum daughter family. But my parents were separated, I consistently was told "your mum did this.. Bla bla bla " from the age of 8/9 then I asked her being told this by a dad loved dearly about a mum I love dearly too made me conflicted and it understand who to trust. When confronted my mum responded "that's a load of crap he did this yanno… Bla bla bla" and so on… I then went through a rollercoaster relationship with my dad and it's resulted in him severely mentally abusing me.

I now am scared to listen or believe any thing any one says no matter how close they are. There's a side to me I don't recognize, I have so much built up frustration and have gone down bad paths to manage it. Alcohol from being 12/13 was my best friend. Then it was boys to older boys that filled the hole I had. Then after that is was self-harm. Running away. I watched as I broke my family. Turned friends against myself calling me "attention seeker" etc. then because I felt my problems weren't enough to be treated with care. I began lying about things but things I felt I had been through (which I hadn't) but I could feel the emotions and live it inside my head like it had happened. Then when I felt so tangled up in these lies I told someone. I was then told I was " evil" "liar" and definitely a "attention seeker"…

I often scare and lose people because talking about everything helps me just get it off my mind. Talking about it to any person helps so much. Someone saying I understand. What you went through was crap. Made me relieved feel good and normal again. But it's caused me to lose people at which I take out on those closest to me and kind of place the blame on them. I try not to but I blank out and it's like another person steps into my body and takes control.

I've often been told even by family to just be happy and get over it and I hope one day people realize that it's not that simple. If you broke your leg and someone told you to just walk, could you? Would you? How would you feel? Bpd as every mental health illness is an illness inside you can't see.

Aimee Wood
Australia

Lost.

Walking through the tunnel,
I'm looking for the light.
Walking slightly left,
And swaying to the right.
I'm lost inside the darkness,
There's nothing here to see.
I hear a thousand people,
But in here it's only me.

I've been walking for so long now,
It's as though it's all I know.
Walking miles at a time,
With still nowhere to go.
One day ill stop walking,
And sit here all alone.
The darkness will comfort me,
Just like me, it's grown.

There is no light to find here,
I finally see it now.
I once had hope id find it,
But I don't remember how.
A child's mind is magic,
I thought there was salvation.
As an adult I've given up,
It just leads to frustration.

Now here I sit in my dark cave,
Of which I can't escape.
The darkness swells inside me,
A spiritual rape.
My punishment brings comfort,
I know I deserve it all.
I built myself up far too high,
One day I had to fall.

Goodbye light and laughter,
You're fondly in my heart.
But now I walk back into the dark,
Why did I ever start?

Jack Mackenzie
UK

Disordered

I am disordered.
I am dis-ordered.
Am I disordered?
Am I dis-ordered?

Am I dis-functioning
Am I dis-arranged

Am I in a state of confusion
Am I in a state of disarray

I am disordered.
I am dis-ordered.

I am Disillusioned.
I am dis- allusioned

What must I do?
I must remember
I must re-member

I need to re-build my world by re-membering who I am by putting back together my-self piece by piece until I feel re-bound to my life and my family.

Only then can I start over. Only then will things change.

Livia Richard
USA

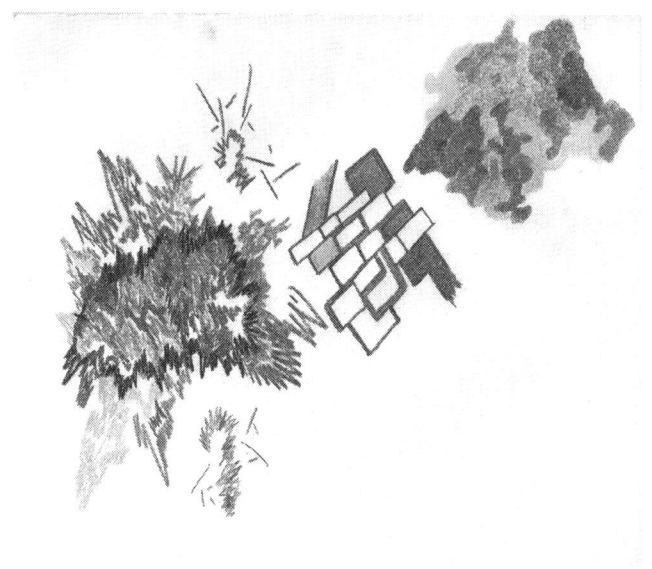

My Brain

Jennifer George
USA

I don't know how much longer I can do this.
But at the same time trying to remind myself
that it's just how I feel right now.
But I also know this feeling will come back
around before too long.
I want off the ride, but I can't get off to please
everyone else.

Stacey Heaney
BPD Survivor
Australia

I've spent the last 14 years wishing I was dead because of bpd. It's a curse. It isn't attention seeking. It's soul destroying. Incredibly painful. It's like a cancer. It eats away at and ruins all that is good about a person. It's a daily fight to keep things in perspective. It's a living hell. It makes you wish you hadn't been born. It's not depression, it's worse than depression because you keep getting your life back, you get so much hope, then you self sabotage everything. It's an evil condition. Those of us who work at trying to understand it and therapy to change.... it's soooo hard

Anonymous
UK

"My thoughts are a NASCAR race at full speed and I am a spectator sitting at the finish line."

Jenifer Purvis
USA

Precariousness means walking on the tightrope and waiting for the fall and, for someone, keeping the balance tastes like an adventure. The feeling that you have to take advantage, that you can only devour - used as you are to fasting, as if you had to stock up before a long famine - prepares the moment of the surrender: daydreamed, foreseen, unavoidable.

Changes, for most people, are scenarios gradually shifting, to which you slowly get used. They are scenes fading from black to white, going through a wide range of colours to perceive, live, study; colours in which you can dive, to which you can get used slowly.

For me, this is more and more rare. The scene change appears to me complete already, all of a sudden, as if everything had happened without me knowing it, overnight, while I was asleep. I wake up and it's all there, ready made. The whole thing falls down on me.

Just only a conversation, a word, a gesture, and everything is suddenly and completely different.

It shakes me.

It influences my mood, my perception of myself and of the outer world, it "changes the structure of the rooms".

I'm the leaf in the wind as usual; I've got no roots. I'm the empty shell; how can I possibly be so evanescent?

I've got no skin. I lack a layer. I'm flawed.

Take care of me. Can't you see I don't work well, I'm broken?
Hold me strong.

I'm endowed with a strong inclination to drama.

When things go wrong, I'm not able to contain the injury and take all the good that can still be taken. No. I go on digging until my nails and fingertips hurt.

A bit of bread, a slice of bread, half a kilogram of bread, a package of biscuits.

A detail out of place, an uncomfortable mattress, a word in the wrong moment, a sleepless night.

I really can't keep my balance, weigh my reactions, think about tomorrow instead of sobering my anger right now.

Moments of different lives succeed in the same day. Different persons, different bodies, as nothing had ever been before the terrible moment I'm living now.

I try to give a meaning to this all, but there's no meaning. One year, two years, ten years... everything could be done in a heartbeat. I recover, then a moment of carelessness is enough and I fall back again. Swollen tummy, headache, 5 o'clock in the morning, chocolate.

It can't be Penelope's shroud forever. It is. Living with this thing means accepting that there will be a few nice moments - spoiled by the anxiety that you must take advantage of them - and many horrible moments when everything will seem impossible to me. I'll wait for my fifteen minutes of glory and then I'll go down again. And I'll already know what will be in store for me. But I'll go on hoping that someday everything will come to an end. And hope is the greatest of evils, the worst possible one. The one that keeps me, that holds me still, the one that should never be there

I stop living.

Then I start again.

Then I fall back

and think that at least I exist.

I'm a leaf in the wind.

Why am I not a free spirit, a racing train,

or a plant, green, standing still on its roots

wherever the wind blows, feeding on sunlight

and nothing else?

A plant on sun and water cannot "binge"

till it feels bad, in order to feel bad,

it takes just what's enough for living

'cause living is its aim.

Why not a film of resin on a tree,

transparent and sheen

idea of freedom?

Why do I suffer as I breath
and as I gaze and as I feel and as I think?

Why can't I think without a noise,

an enormous noise,

like a troublesome

and obsessive, haunting buzz

(a doom)?

Eleonora Nappi
Italy
Translated by Blandina Comenale Pinto
(with contributions from Ombretta and Eleonora)

Wednesday's Child

She doesn't want narrative today. Slices of pure lyricism shortcut from brain to skin without waiting for the words to form, a free association of mind and body that will leave scars she won't want to explain.

You're supposed to have grown out of this girl, remember? You're supposed to be bigger than both of us now.

Feelings drift like blind men's fingers, seeking out every crack and wrinkle in the day, raw skin scraping on concrete and sand, bones aching with years-worth of cold. Sleeping on rocks and under bridges, it became second nature to make herself scarce whenever she was not welcome. She became adept at moving on.

But today is not one of those second nature days. Today she shuffles, stumbles on her own belatedness, the things she passed up, the things that pass her by. Knows that she still doesn't know anything. Wonders if wisdom is worth the price.

Just keep walking. Tears can form and spill and dry. No one will notice. Just keep your head down.

Or wipe it all clean. Lie down on the tracks. Fall asleep in the snow. Let your foot slip at the top of the ravine. Lean a little further over, spread out your arms, just let it all go.

What did I say to you last time, girl? Your life shouldn't hang on the colour of the sky.

And she knows that these little things shouldn't be so urgent, but sometimes a smile - or no smile, or silence - is all the difference it takes for the sun to come out in her head. And she knows that it was never going to be easy, but sometimes she just wants to let it all slide...

And I know I'll have to go find her again, sitting out on another park bench in the cold, singing to herself as the light fades away and the bottle goes from half full to almost empty, and the blood dries, and the people skirt round her thinking she's crazy.

It will be me that holds her. Me that holds her in, holds up the mirror, makes her smile to see herself after all these years still running away from home. And me that takes her back to yet another bed instead of that park bench, makes sure she brushes her teeth and changes out of her clothes, sets her alarm for another morning. Me that tucks her in at night, with the extra blanket she wouldn't fetch for herself, and sings her back to sleep at 1 a.m. after the ghost-trains wake her up with their howling.

And me at last who makes a tale of it all, when she doesn't want words and the songs dry up inside her, when she feels so hollow she could just blow away.

I am the guardian of my solitude. Tomorrow we'll have a long way to go.

The rest is silence. For today.

Libby Boyd
Thailand

Imprisonment of Thoughts

I'm uneasy
Feeling queasy
Shaking, quaking
Exasperating
I'm worn down
Can't hold my ground
My head's spinning
Confidence thinning
Everything's unraveling
I feel myself traveling
Down the same road
My wellbeing erodes
Prisoner of thoughts
My stomach is in knots
On the verge of tears
I'm being consumed by all of my fears
I don't know how I'll make it through
When my insides are coming unglued
Please just make it stop!
My heart's beating so fast, it's going to pop!
I'm sweating
Constantly fretting
Existence
I think I need some assistance
I'm paranoid
Now I tend to avoid
Almost everyone
I've succumbed
To unhealthy thinking
It's hard not to do when you're sinking
Now I swallow my pride
And realize I'm just along for the ride
Maybe someday things will be different
Until then, better get used to the imprisonment

Shawnna Hastings-Downey
Canada

Masks

Eyes stinging from tears she fights to hold back,
as yet again the Mask must be put back on.
That loathsome Mask!
Burning from the inside out.
Heightening all the pain and sorrow until you don't
feel anything anymore.
Only to have it triggered over and over again.
Yet no one realizes the anguish she has to endure;
they can't see through the Mask's fog.

"Be Strong!" "Be Happy!" "Deal with it!"

So many things easily said and stated.
Yet for someone as fragile as her, not so easy.
Lost, not knowing who she really is.
Raw from the constant inner turmoil, she feels
completely alone.
The Mask she wears is unwillingly her only constant
companion.
Those able to glimpse through and crack her hated
Mask she keeps close to her Heart.
Loving them unconditionally.
Leaving herself open to heartache and pain.

Having to watch those she loves walk or even run
away with a piece of her Heart seems far too often.
Some so cruelly, sneakily and intentionally.
While still others; don't realize, intend or want to.
Never, it seems, able to grieve fully.
Or the right way.
For the Mask is never far away.
Always waiting around for the smell of un-shed tears.
Or the feeling of pressure coming from her heavy
Heart;
ready to take it's place.

Star Williams
USA

Snapshots:

Everything ends. You either do it until you die or it leaves. The choice you make it how you cope with the end, and how long you prolong the inevitable. It isn't about denying the end; it's about avoiding it. You run from commitments knowing you'll ruin them prematurely. Only you last until death. Everything else leaves.

"You can have a disagreement without fighting," He says. I stare blankly, tears rolling down my face.

"I understand that, but it doesn't sound right."

We're fighting because he asked me to carry bags upstairs that I thought were too heavy. I've been yelling about problems I'm probably making up for five minutes.

"I think I'm going to go."

"You can't leave me."

"I'm just going home."

"I'm never going to see you again! You're mad at me, you'll be mad at me forever."

"You know that's not true."

I say ok but the tears pour out harder. I turn around and try to gather them. This is weakness. This is the part of me that is unlovable. I can't let it be seen.

"Fine." He sighs and sits back down. I'm overwhelmingly guilty. I've been told this is emotional manipulation. I don't understand that. All evidence points to the fact that when people leave they don't come back.

~

My emotions are a tornado. It is impossible to distinguish one from another. If I feel one feeling I am feeling them all. Happiness is sadness is anger. I react to all emotions the same. I push them away. Feelings are uncomfortable and are ultimately not worth it. You get nothing out of emotions, just more of them.

"How do you feel?"

I'm sitting on a couch. A woman with motherly eyes looks at me from a parallel couch.

I can't think of an answer. I feel. If I feel one emotion I feel them all. I am a sith lord. Sadness becomes fear becomes anger becomes manic joy. I wonder what it's like to feel one thing. To be able to have control. These are all the things I think.

"I'm ok."

It's not a lie. I'm what I call ok. Something eating away inside me, crawling out through my tear ducts.

"I'm ok."

~

I'm terrified of conflict. People don't get unmad. They're mad at you forever. I don't have a very good perception of time. Things only happen right now or last forever. Neutrality is better.

"Did you ever want an apology from me?"

The beginning asking for an end. We're sitting in a car. I would like to not be. The trees and cars suddenly don't seem real. None of it does. Everything melts away and I don't know how long I've been sitting in silence.

I don't know what to say. Yes? Do I dare take the out? Do I dare ask for what I want? Do I dare?

"I think we're good."

~

Other people have feelings. I know this is a fact. I forget that. Everyone's top motivation is clearly to cause me harm, I feel that. I want everyone to take my feelings into consideration, but I can't do the same for them.

"You have really negative energy. I'm not the only one who notices"

I sincerely don't care. This wasn't my fault. I throw it back.

"Because you never pay attention to me! I'm not important to you."

"I live with you don't I?"

"Barely."

"That makes no sense."

That makes no sense. I feel it, so it must be true. How does everyone not feel this? How does no one feel what I'm feeling. Why am I alone?

"That makes no sense."

~

I like swimming. Swimming feels like thinking but easier. Rushing through, meeting resistance, blurry, stinging. There's a chance you may not resurface. There's a chance this will be the last time.

My head is on fire. It's very loud. I'm struggling to breathe. I pick up a piece of fruit. I hear screaming.

I see a picture of myself on the wall. It disgusts me. I take it down. I remove all evidence of myself from the house. I'm the first-born. There are a lot.

"Why did you do that?" She asks.
"I didn't want to look at myself."
"Why?"
"Everything's my fault. I can't do anything right."
"Was 9/11 your fault?"
This was extreme. But I am not wrong.
"I don't know. Probably,"
"It's just puberty." She puts the pictures back up.
~

I am garbage person. It's an endearing nickname I created for myself. It lets me off the hook. I can't be held responsible for my actions. They are inevitable. I am garbage person.

"I don't want to date you" I say. "I like you too much."

What I mean is I wouldn't want to subject you to the emotional nonsense that is dating me. I see myself screaming at you, lying to you, cheating on you, blaming you.
"I'm not a good person."
"I know what you mean." You flick your cigarette.
"No you don't." We kiss.
"I don't want to date you."
~
I should be ashamed of myself, and I am. I'd call myself an opportunist if I had any objective. I romanticize qualities in others I cannot find in myself. I lie selfishly. It is always to protect myself. I am a coward.

"What are you writing?"
"A story."

Kat Kaplan
USA

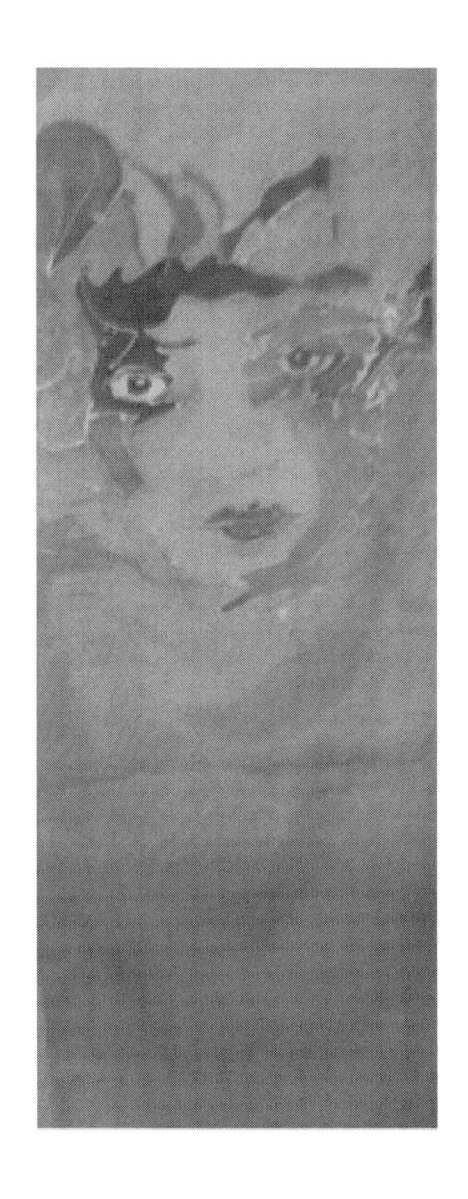

Untitled

Tee Taylor
UK

Who are you?
You weren't here yesterday.
Didn't need plasters yesterday .
That person knew herself.
I think.
I liked her . I think .
She seemed confident , funny.
People probably don't like that though .
No one has replied to me all morning .
 I was too confident yesterday .
They hate me ,
probably together right now happy to be away from overbearing me,
Screw everyone.
I will never be loved for me anyway by these so called family and friends.
I do so much for others .
Unless I'm truly selfish maybe but don't see it.
How can I start afresh and get people to like me again.
Probably too late.
God I'm so awful.
Ooh big sis wants to go for lunch .
My life is fabulous.
I think

Charlotte Mathews
UK

Honestly

Happy. It's been a pretty good day. I'm so tired though. I always am.

"Are you mad at me? You just seem mad at me." No sorry, that's just... My face. I'm actually fine. I'm ok...

I think.

Oh god, his face.
Say something!
He looks so sad.
Why do you ALWAYS do this?
You can't just be normal.

My stomach dropped,
Guilt...

I think.

He'll get sick of me eventually.
Everyone does.

Fear...
Guilt...

I feel sick
I could just run away
I should probably just kill myself

Anger...

I hate myself for even thinking it.
We've been here.
I've run away before but I was the problem.
I can't just die, because that's too final.

Guilt...
Fear...

Anger...
Fear...

Fuck.

And then there's nothing.
Look at his face... SAY SOMETHING!

"I'm just tired, honestly."

Sinead Hope-Brown
England

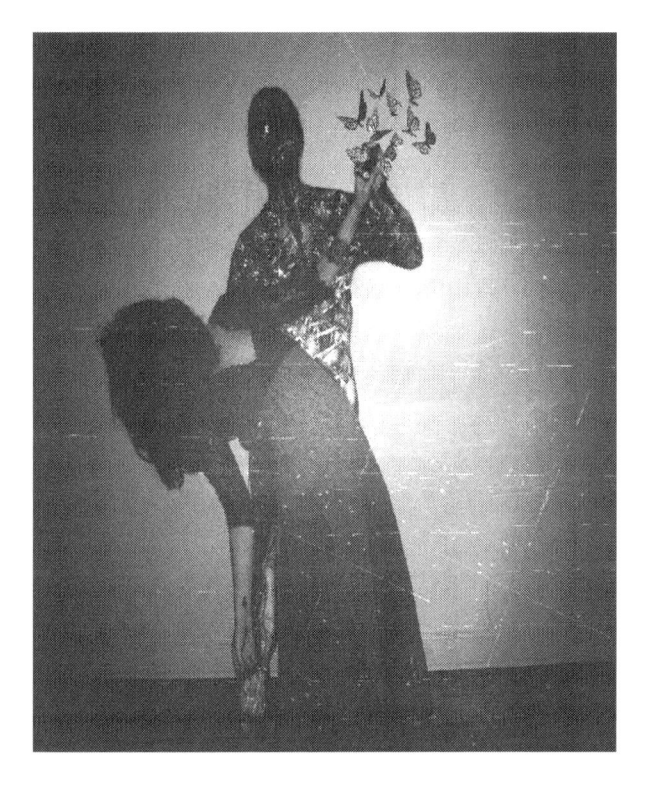

**"If I can't rid you, then I will learn to live with you.
& that is my freedom~"**

Liliana Beth Reckless
Canada

Darkness surrounds me,
It engulfs me in fear,
Wherever I go,
The darkness is near

Kirsty McCarthy
Wales

I have a tendency to assume my friends opinions of me (that they pity me and my sad little life) so I end up resenting them and pushing them away even though they've not done anything wrong. I spend most of my time angry at so many people for no reason.

Colleen Clothier
UK

No one is all bad or all good however our choices speak to our character therefore I suggest that:
~ if we want to be understood, we show understanding
~ if we want to be respected, we show respect
~ if we want to be loved, we show each other love
~ if we want to be forgiven, we ourselves practice forgiveness

Tania Neilson
Australia

She's a broken girl
But she's got a lot to give
Got a lot of soul
And heart
Deep down
And she falls over her self
She feels her greatness
But tears it apart
Wants to live in the sun
But made a home in the dark
Gives all that she has
To the things that go no where
But she wants to live
She knows she's beautiful
She knows she's worth it
Believes In good and still knows evil

Feeling so defective
Doesn't even move"

Alexandria Hutson
USA

I'm having one of those days where you question everything and don't know if you're coming or going or how to fix the causalities in my life as a result of my illness. So much is going wrong at once and it's hard to keep level headed to think of solutions.

I'm sure they'll come when they are meant to while at the same time thinking maybe I don't deserve it, maybe this is as good as it gets for me. I feel lonely yet I can't consider a relationship. Who would be bothered to put up with it?
Who should have to?

Stacey Heaney
BPD Survivor
Australia

The Beast in Me

It seems strange to me that for some people, today is just like any other day. Waking up to the same sky, the same noises, sipping the same cup of tea.

Today, for me is not like any other day. Today I wake up with my head running a million miles an hour. No matter how many spanners I try to throw into the spinning wheels, the cogs keep on turning. I can feel the grind in my head and I'm all too aware that if the noise continues, the beast inside me will stir.

She's always there, lurking in the background, reminding me that what goes up, must come down. Today I feel her tired eyes beginning to open. Though her lids are heavy, she fights the goodness that I am trying to latch on to, but she is stubborn and without reason her eyes fly open like a tired child refusing to sleep.

She has been paying me visits more often these days. She drags my racing heart into my throat and I feel my insides explode. My lungs no longer serve their purpose and my ribs crack open and fall into my stomach, the sharp ends piercing me like shrapnel. The heat rises from my throat and the blood stains my cheeks, my face, and it pools behind my eyes. Rising up like a tidal wave and rolling down my back, straight to my finger tips. The blood rises endlessly and I drown in the knowledge that not one person on this earth can anchor me down. In the end, I always find myself sailing away.

The beast is a part of me and I know she will howl through the days and nights and eventually cry herself to sleep. I am ashamed that the beast has been woken but this time my fingers won't stop writing because I think perhaps somewhere out there are people with their own beasts wreaking havoc, just like mine.

I feel tired. I feel sad. I feel everything. My skin is so thin that the innocent words of others burn holes right through me. I feel like I have exhausted my own words though. That they have been said too many times and the people who love me don't deserve to hear them anymore. I don't want to take any passengers with me on this ride because I know they eventually tire of me after I've beaten them down and they timidly ask to get off. I know this because it happens all too often, so I use every ounce of strength to keep the beast at bay until I am alone and no one can see just how ugly I can be. It is here that I set her free and as I watch her flying above my head she swoops down, ripping apart my old scars and puncturing my insides until I no longer resemble a human being.

I hang my head and I let myself be flooded with grief. Who will love me after I have introduced them to the monster inside? I smart from so many broken promises of safety and somewhere to call home. I remember the innocent, unknowing voices speaking of growing old and making our grass the greenest of all. What they didn't realise was, there was never any grass there to begin with. Just a pile of dirt. A graveyard, where I have buried the pieces of me that I don't want to remember.

Monique Potter
Australia

Save me St Jude (patron saint of the hopeless)

Feeling like the ground has fallen out from under me again. Things just started to pick up: signs of light at the end of the tunnel, but just over a week has past and and my world is in complete darkness again. Pitch black. I've cried until my tears have run dry. I numbed myself with alcohol and sex with my boyfriend. Now I'm deflated; pretending to fain interest in my boyfriend's story about his neighbor's son borrowing his Harley to get to work tomorrow. I make noises at the appropriate intervals to hide the fact that I couldn't be less interested. All I can think about is that I'm out of distractions, my boyfriend is about to go to sleep and I have several hours of insomnia ahead of me which will consist of the horrible memory of the events of the day consuming my thoughts causing my heart to ache and creating a sickening churning in my stomach that feels like the physical manifestation of utter dread. I feel so alone in my pain. The few that know my suffering feel sorry for me but their empathy unfortunately doesn't change a thing and therefore offers no comfort. They cannot protect me from this. So back to; sleepless nights, anxiety, inability to eat, depression, emptiness and thoughts of suicide for me. The worst part is feeling obliged to pretend I am coping; plastering on a smile so that I don't cause the ones I love pain by allowing them to see I'm really dying inside. I am paralyzed by feelings of total lack of control. I believe that feeling powerless makes people feel hopelessness and I believe hopeless is the most dangerous of emotions. Without hope there is nothing. It makes justifying existence extremely difficult

Tania Neilson
Australia

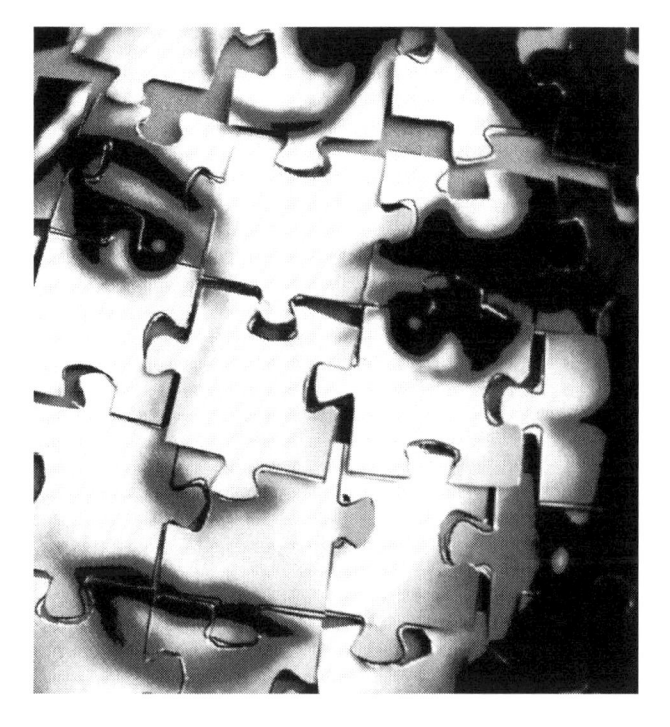

Pieces of Me

Melanie Carrillo
USA

My mind and me.

My mind is broken,
a little bent
Needs to let off steam
But has no vent.

I've tried plasters and pills,
And potions and lotions
I've tried old wife's tales
And other such notions

What is this emotion that I feel,
Is it fake or is it real?
I get so confused and get in such a muddle
That it makes me melt into an emotional puddle.

Sometimes it's like my brain just farts
Or gets a little better then reboots right from the start.
Sometimes I'm awake but my minds stays asleep.
Sometime it wanders off and plays hide and seek.

It lies and tricks me like I'm one big joke
It suffocates me so I emotionally choke.
Doctors and shrinks think they have a cure
My mind just laughs and says "yes sure!"

I don't have any wounds or scars you can see
But it's all very real and scary to me.
I have to explain my self again and again
For this mind I've been given that refuses to mend

Sometimes I can't think so very straight,
It's hard for me to concentrate,
Sometimes I forget.....now what was I going to say?
It's a constant battle every single day,

Sometimes it likes me to go wild
Sometimes it wants me to act like a child,
Sometimes it wants to hide away,
Sometimes it wants to come out and play.

It's full of constant ups and downs
Fake smiles and endless frowns,

So the next year of my life went as follows, relationship break down.... I blamed it on living at my mum's.... So we decided to get out own place once again....

I was then on one serious downward spiral I became really low. I would just randomly burst into tears I didn't know why. I would randomly cause arguments with my other half without knowing really why. I would end up at my mum's twice a week.

I found this website I started off going on it to escape the real world, and real people thing is it was like a chat site met the Sims you had your own avatars you talk to people all over the world. It was a great escape... Problem is I found it more fun and better being someone else in a different life where people didn't know what I looked like or my problems! I found myself being sucked into the cyber world more and more I ended up spending 18 hours a day online! It felt so good I didn't care that the house was a mess that I hadn't been outside in weeks although I lived with my partner I didn't sleep with him, in the same bed as him or even talk to him.....

Claire Lou
UK

This one's about being numb...

You say explain to me what it's like to feel numb?
Ok here goes

There I am done...
Kirsty McCarthy
Wales

Sea of misery.

Stare into my eyes and tell me what you see. Is it black and forlorn and distraught before me? Is your mind still shinning brightly for you? Mine is bleak and cares nothing of what I do.
Your eyes are looking for distractions. So you can't see mine and their lack of satisfaction.

Please tell me why this is as it is.

Why are your eyes alive and mine dead? Why do yours look to care and mine look to dread? Your world is solid like the hard wood of the trees. Mine, well mine has drifted apart with the breeze.
You try to help me, even though I can't help but to plead. Perhaps one day I shall understand and my body will cease to bleed. Patience is the key; let your mind know I care. Tell your eyes to keep looking, even into the insanity and despair.

Embrace the darkness which has already come for me. But stay away and your mind shall be free. Your mind understands for me you must cry. Whereas mine simply wishes I would die.
Your mind is bright, mine is not.

There is no darkness in you, only that bright light. Darkness and fears are all I have in my eternal night. You have pain but I have pain without boundaries. Pain is my pleasure, you get used to it I suppose; a few more tears build up and you're good to go.
You must stay away and always stay bright. Me, I'll always be like the night. Do not try to understand, you will get lost in the sea.
A sea of pain, torment and day-to-day misery.

-ScHarna

Truth is, underneath it all, I'm just a frightened little girl... lost along the path to my own destruction.

I have no one to blame for my fears but myself- I let them in. I let them all in. I let them stay.

They became so overpowering and attached that they never want to leave.

I wish they knew how unwelcome they were, and still are...
since they got here, they do nothing except tear away at every part of me that wants normality (whatever that is) and they pull away at my insides, poking, prodding, piercing; bleeding me dry. Dry of every last molecule of trust, and faith and belief that I may try to hold in anything or anyone in my world around me...

The fears leave me lonely... well, almost... you see, my fears have family... they came to visit not long after the fears arrived and got themselves well and truly settled. I wish i never let them in... i should have told them "Sorry, no vacancies"... Upon check-in i asked their names...One replied Anxiety, the other one, Depression... And how very exciting, (not) they were expecting their first child- Borerline Personality Disorder...

I hated the day they all decided to stay...
Because now they're here, I don't know how to get them to leave.

The house is full... but the home is empty... and that's one of the worst feelings in the world...

Courtney Cornall
Western Australia

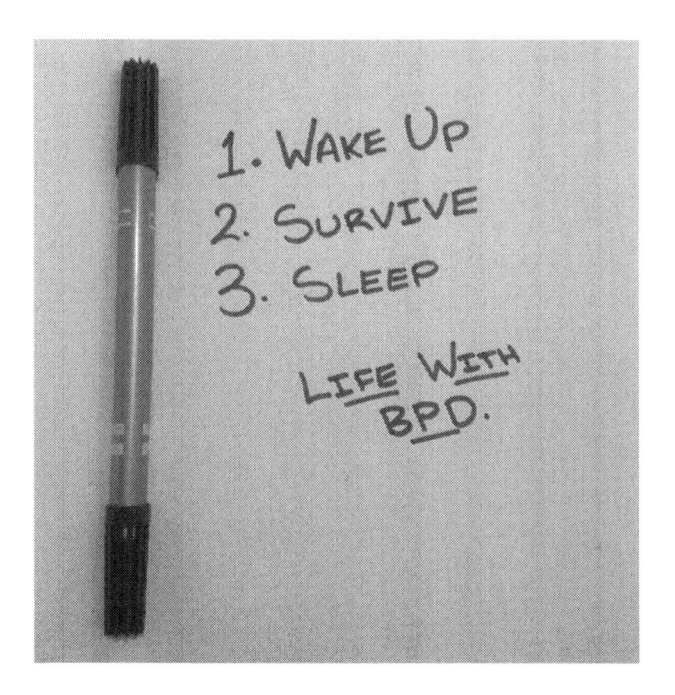

Life with BPD

Hayley Figiel.
England

All in my Head

Everyday is a challenge
Everyday is a struggle
I'm left here to scavenge
Rummaging through the rubble
Trying to piece together
My broken heart
With how much I endeavor,
It seems like an art
Constantly fooling everyone
I don't want them to see
How much damage has been done
To the real me
Everything is a game
And I always wear masks
Avoiding the shame
Is the hardest of tasks
I've never felt good enough
Or strong like they said
The going's always been rough
Or was that all in my head?

Shawnna Hastings-Downey
Canada

Remembering On My Own

I am not sure who I am writing this to. Perhaps myself. Perhaps to you. Perhaps to no one at all. Everyone is moving on. The world is moving on. It turns and turns without me, spinning on its axis as it has done for billions of years. I am drifting in the wake of my own big bang. I am stranded in time. I'm breathing what was long-ago and merely existing in the future. My body floats above everyone and my insides hide away in a crevice of the past. I am smiling and hoping for everything to end. I am deleting history. I am handing out the last rose. I am lying in the sun, the white sheet beneath my burning body. I'm searching for someone who can fill the gaps. I find someone and dig a hole. I love someone, I dig deeper. I still love. I miss her in spite of myself. I hate her. I love her. I love and hate everything that she is, and I leave all the same. A glass of cheap wine spills on my words. They remained stained as I sang the song of New York that reminded me of a new memory I made and I wish I never had. I bring all I can. I do all I can. Consciousness. A wise mind. I look up my symptoms and shake my head. What sort of life is this. I question my fight. I am standing at the lights and I step out as close to the curb as I dare and I dream. It is only a dream, but who else can understand these words? What do I believe in? I come to this office, full of suits, the colour of someone's demise, the pin stripes pointing straight to hell. I am ashamed. Ashamed of this weakness that I have. Ashamed that my strength wanes and disappears from time to time, disappears from under my eyelids, gone from beneath me. Swept up and begging it to be handed to the first person who passes me by. A swapping of souls, even if it's just for a moment.

I am out of luck. Out of my mind. Dying to exchange my memories for something tedious. A memory that leaves no tracks in the earth. My memories; an earth mover, scraping giant holes in the past. Blind me and save me from falling into those shallow graves. A hole dug for each recollection. I have almost exhausted my last spark. You have walked these halls with me. You have seen the murky corridors of my mind. You have been a witness to the waves that threw me from my ledge, even when you weren't really there at all, you were treading my path.

Memories, on purpose made. The soles of my shoes are worn, like everything that lies beneath me. You have prepared a new future. I wear my old skin like a Queen wears her crown. Unasked for and impossible to shed. Do not pity me, nor forget me. I am opening up my heart without any fear of breach. An unconditional understanding that flows from one fingertip to the other. The days creep up slowly and turn into the very hour where it seems all of this began. The colours are just as vivid as they were 3 years ago. The smells and the sounds wash over me like a tidal wave and take me back to another time. Another life. Another me. A layer of dust has settled over this bright landscape and it lies in waiting like a dormant volcano begging to erupt, dying to break the peace and the sanity that I thought I once had a firm hold of. The days churn by like a dream. I am a sleepwalker. A child. A living ghost. A shadow of the past, a splinter of the present and a strained breath of the future. I tried to find a way to put the dust back together, but it wasn't to be. I tried in so many ways, but each time, the dust crumbled in my shaking hands and fell back to the earth. I tried to hide the dust. Hide it away in spaces that no one would ever think to look. But it crept out, one piece at a time until it lay at my feet once again. I scatter the dust over my ocean of sins, like a fallen soldier, unaware of the penitence she should be owning if her flesh were to prevail. On my doorstep the sacrilege still burns holes in my skin. I want to rip up the past and flush it away with as much dignity as a dead goldfish. But it is more deserving than that and just not that easy. The past seems to lie ahead of me instead. The past becomes my future. It spreads out in front of me like a burnt harvest. I wade through the dying embers, praying for the strength to endure the remaining flames that lick at my feet like diminutive devils imploring me to burn below the earths crust. Though the worst is over, the aftermath remains colossal and I am treading upon broken boards. I measure and calculate each step, treading as softly as I can so as not to wake the dead. As I soak up this dying harvest, I breathe in the smoke, knowing that it will clear, but uncertain of when or how. The next steps I take are most precarious. Life hangs in the balance and it is all too soon. I delete myself from the world as it exists and shield myself from the blinding light that burns my translucent skin, like a helpless ant melting through a magnifying glass by a child's lack of conscience. I need to bow out for awhile and remind myself how it feels to breathe. I need to remove myself from the hurt that people cause me unintentionally, because it floods my mind again and brings back that familiar ache that only I can make disappear. Live your life to the fullest. Love with all your heart. Be honest and kind but never forget the past. There is no blame. No guilt. The past is a lesson and we must shoulder the burden to make us better people. Will you stand with me awhile and remember, because it hurts too much to remember on my own.

Monique Potter
Australia

When you suffer from unfitness you feel unsuitable even in your own illness. You long to be more unfit in order to outstand at least in that, you want to go down and down in order to be the best in denying life. Yes, when you suffer from unfitness you end up in the paradox for which you feel less than those who are able to deny life better than you do.

When you suffer from unfitness there's no context in which you can feel safe, because your illness takes the shape of any situation and place that you touch, and settles in there as if that place or situation has always been its home.

When you suffer from unfitness, in my opinion, you start suffering as a child, when something or somebody has maybe marked your forehead with some original flaw.

When you suffer from unfitness, I think, you never recover. The most evident wounds are replaced by faded scars, and the whole thing is less stagy, less showy, less loud, but it remains like a warning, colouring all adjectives with a hue of excess or defect, and leaving an unbridgeable gap between what you are and what you feel you must be.

When you suffer from unfitness "you perceive everything that happens", even before it happens, like the dogs who can feel the thunder before the storm. Sometimes, it may be that you perceive things that don't actually happen, too.

But when you suffer from unfitness "you have nothing", and you go on and on looking for what is not there, regardless of what is actually there. Because it's an unconditioned reflex, a manufacturing defect, the unhealthy habit of revolving around oneself. A canker bound to go deeper and deeper in time.

Eleonora Nappi
Italy
Translated by Blandina Comenale Pinto

Behind the Clouds: Living with BPD

One line is all it takes to fill my head with noises I don't want to hear,
They speak over and over, telling me things,
Filling me with anger, dread and fear.
Sadness then takes over. The darkness not long to follow.

And then soon all people see is me,
Unable to keep my once able head up,
Tears and sadness swallowing me.

I feel like I am always fighting – life, myself, everyone,
Just to get through every day.
And it makes me angry that other people put in half the effort,
And they get to be happy, and I'm only OK.

They say this illness will go away.
Or it will kill me.
Sometimes I don't know which.

From the time I open my eyes in the morning I live in fear of it Taking over me,
What lies behind the clouds of the day?
The trick is this –
Is there a beautiful sun that will create the most amazing stunning day or a thunderstorm with a severe weather warning waiting for me?

Many days there is both.
Many days there is one.
Sometimes I stay in bed and never know.

I have been given the tools to make most days good and fewer days bad,
But what I think someone with BPD really wants,
Is just for someone to stay around, take away the sad,
And be strong when we're being mad.

And love.
Everyone needs love.
A nightmare and perfect dream at the same time.

Strength I am finding though, however, slowly, can be found in me.
Each day I see the clouds part means I am prepared to do battle with another day.
And love, however dangerous, I have found hidden in the depths of BPD.
Each day, each hour, I am here means I do and can love me and those around me.

I have BPD.
I am stronger than I know.
There is even love everywhere in my life – even in my illness. Sometimes it is just hard to see it behind the clouds.

Mel Wilson
Australia

Waiting to fall –
BPD and obsessive attachments

[The quotes at the beginning of each Part of this post, are from 'The Buddha and the Borderline' by Kiera Van Gelder.]

Part I – What

"Of the three poisons that obstruct the mind's clarity…..attachment is the most difficult of the afflictions. You have to be constantly vigilant, or it will take over your mind."

Sometimes I wonder what love feels like. What it feels like for other people, and how they would describe it. Some people say that 'love is not a feeling', by which they mean that love is a matter of the head as well as the heart, and that feelings must be backed up by actions, or at least be consistent with one's actions, otherwise love is just an empty four-letter word.

So often, love feels like an empty four-letter feeling. When I try and cast my heart-eye inward, to try and pinpoint what it feels like, it's as if I'm searching in the dark, groping for something utterly elusive. Sometimes that disturbs me. At other times, I convince myself that it's just a question of a perfectly natural inability to describe the indescribable. That it's not a question of some deep flaw within me. And yet –

I can tell you with absolute clarity what obsessive love (or attachment) feels like. It's almost as if the quality of reality itself is dependent upon the intensity of obsession – if a feeling is not completely overwhelming me and taking me over, then it's as if I'm not feeling it at all. In a way that is very hard to describe, it's as if I know there is a feeling there, but I'm not quite sensing it. I feel it – but I don't feel it. Maybe it's just a matter of terminology – maybe there's no actual difference between the two.

Or it could be that the difficulty stems from the calibration of my emotions. On my emotional Richter scale, the magnitude ten earthquakes completely overshadow the magnitude four tremors. It's as if having been exposed to the thumping bass sounds of music at full volume, my senses have lost the ability to hear a full range of sounds. Intense emotions drown out all other music – I can feel the vibrations, but I cannot hear the melody. The opposite of intensity feels like emptiness – even when there's something there.

Part II – How

"As soon as I'm touched, all of my power drains away and I'll become a supplicant again."

In my own drama of obsessive love, there are two players – The One Who Chases, and The One Who Falls. I think and feel very differently about them. I despise the game playing of the first, and am moved by the vulnerability of the second. I don't want to accept the former, but I'd like to hold the latter in my arms. I suspect my therapist would tell me that the 'two' are just one little girl, looking for something that is missing. That I'm 'splitting' her out into all-bad and all-good. In which case, I ultimately have to either disown them both or embrace them both together.

The initial stages of a relationship are heady for many people, and the excitement of the 'chase', or the thrill of the flirtation, is intoxicating. I don't think there is anything unusual in that. But for me, there is an incredibly addictive quality to those feelings. I can't imagine a more powerful drug, or a more potent high. I wish that I could plug you in to how it feels, when I'm in the grip of that rush. I wish that I hook you up to my IV, so that whatever's flowing through my veins, could flow through yours too. If I imagine it, it looks like liquid gold. If I sense it with my eyes closed, it feels like bundles of electricity bouncing around inside me, trying to get out. It's a whirlwind of breathless expectation and thought in action, all swirling around

a centre of powerful invincibility. The perfect storm. The perfect calm.
I flit from one thought to another – I am all over the place, but also just in one place. The place of this feeling, here and now, over-riding everything else. I see with perfect clarity. I shut my eyes to feel a little deeper. Rational mind slowly recedes and the focus of my inner mind narrows down to the width of a pin. I shut my eyes, and it feels like I'm standing at the top of a rollercoaster, about to jump on and join the ride. It feels like I'm waiting to fall.

The 'falling' happens when I'm not watching. Before I know it I'm caught in the grip of something just as intense, and just as addictive. There is nothing exciting or euphoric about this phase of obsessive love. It is horribly painful, and it is all-consuming. The One Who Chases is under the illusion that she is powerful and in control, although I know that that's a lie. But the illusion gives her strength, and allows her to revel in the chase. The One Who Falls knows that she is powerless and helpless; that she is in the grip of something, and someone, that she cannot control. She is at the mercy of her intense emotions, and The One Who Chases has abandoned her to them, defenceless and alone.

When I'm in this phase of an obsessive attachment, the other person becomes my entire world. They are my first thought upon waking, and my last thought at night. They are a place (either in reality, or in my head) that I escape to constantly and willingly, losing myself in every conceivable way. As desperately as The One Who Chases wants to take someone else over, the One Who Falls wants to be entirely taken over and engulfed by the object of her attachment. This phase of obsessive love is so painful because although I idealise the centre of my universe, they are always only human, and always just beyond my reach. Connectedness feels only ever partial, and my neediness is like a well that just gets deeper, the more I try and fill it.

Apart from a need for intensity, the One Who Chases and The One Who Falls have one other thing in common. They both long to be touched. The One Who Falls wants to be touched in order to feel loved. The One Who Chases wants to be touched in order to feel alive. And that is her undoing. Her illusion of control unravels, and she has to leave the stage. A single touch can floor her, but it's The One Who Falls who ends up in a heap, horrified at the spotlight thrown upon her need.

Part III – Why

"Why does this always happen? .....it's a reflection of some sort of deep trouble – a desire that eclipses reason and takes me over…"

It's very easy to judge ourselves for our obsessive attachments, and to hate ourselves for them, particularly as they can lead us to behave in ways that we may consider to be 'out of character' or even 'wrong'. Sometimes, despite the pain, it feels that there is a certain beauty to obsessive love. It feels self-sacrificial in its other-centred-ness. Love is often described in personified terms –'love is patient', 'love is kind'. But although obsessive love can feel self-sacrificial, it's more like a force, than a person. And as a force, the darker side of it can sometimes be devoid both of reason, and of morality. It's not that obsessive love chooses 'wrong' over 'right' – it's just that in a world taken over entirely by the object at its centre, nothing else seems to matter.

But rather than judging myself for my obsessive attachments, I am trying to figure out what they can teach me. Rather than trying to find the fault within myself, I am trying to find the explanation. Let me be clear – I am not trying to whitewash painful situations or make excuses for hurtful behaviour. But there is a reason (or a multiplicity of reasons), for our obsessive relationships. This is not just 'the way we are', where 'the the way we are' is an indirect way of saying 'broken – cannot be mended'. For me, I think obsessive relationships are about two things. They are about what was missing, or what became twisted, in terms of childhood attachments. But they are also a coping strategy.

More than one therapist has suggested to me that my obsessive relationships were a way of coping with life. It seemed an odd idea at first, but looking back, the truth of that explanation is obvious. Those relationships, whether 'in my head', or played out in reality, all occurred at particularly difficult or dark times for me. They were an escape, they took me (mentally) out of the situation I was in, and they gave me something else to immerse myself in. They were a distraction of the most powerful kind. I used to wonder why I only started self-harming a couple of years ago, until a therapist once again suggested that it was because I was replacing one coping mechanism with another. Obsessional relationships may have been a 'readily available' coping strategy in the past, but given changes in circumstances, such as working, and being a wife and mother, they could no longer operate in the same way.

A friend of mine recently gave me an incredibly helpful way of describing what is going on with me, in situations when I might otherwise be tempted to judge myself. She said that I was 'processing something'. It seems to me that that is a much kinder way to talk about the patterns of obsessional relationships that we can fall into, while also motivating us to try and discover what is really going on.
'Processing' can mean so many things. It can mean becoming obsessed with your best friend; it can mean having an internet flirtation with someone you barely know; it can mean 'falling in love' with someone in a position of power. And sometimes, it can mean inappropriately trying to push boundaries with someone that you are just starting to trust. I have been so busy keeping watch on The One Who Falls, and guarding against the possibility of developing feelings of obsessive love in the context of my current therapy, that I didn't even notice when The One Who Falls opened the door for The One Who Chases to come out and play. On the one hand, I want to lock her

away keep her behind closed doors. On the other hand, I know that there could be no safer environment for her to play in. No other place in which she can be herself, without fear of condemnation, or without risk of causing long-term hurt to others or to herself.

So in the name of 'processing', as deeply uncomfortable as it may feel – let the games begin.

Clara Bridges
UK

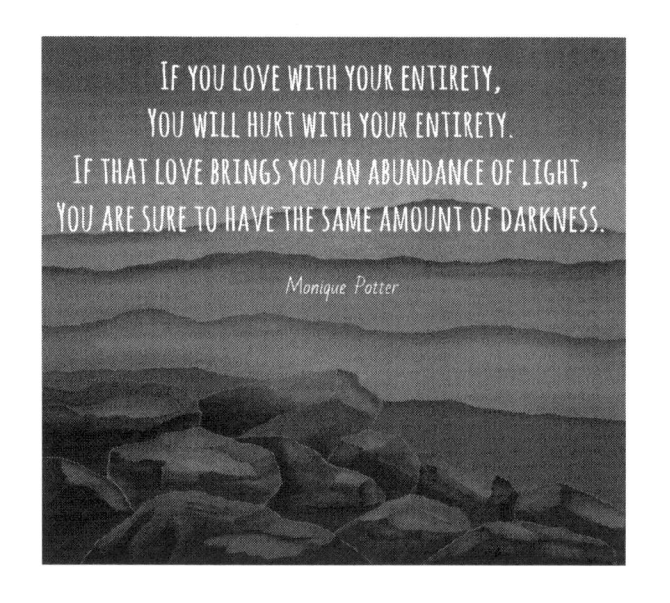

> IF YOU LOVE WITH YOUR ENTIRETY,
> YOU WILL HURT WITH YOUR ENTIRETY.
> IF THAT LOVE BRINGS YOU AN ABUNDANCE OF LIGHT,
> YOU ARE SURE TO HAVE THE SAME AMOUNT OF DARKNESS.
>
> Monique Potter

Words

Saadh Kent
Australia

II.

Relationships

They say we "accept the love we think we deserve" and this is exactly why I struggle to balance my BPD and my relationship. I absolutely love and trust him, but my BPD doesn't. I try to remind myself that he will never do anything to purposely hurt me and that he loves me more than anything in the world, but somehow I find myself back where I started and then that's it, it's taken over. I do not understand why he would want me or love me so I start believing that he's lying or going to betray me... That he will leave me and I won't be able to cope. I am terrified of life without him but terrified of life with him. I know I will push him away if this carries on, but I cannot shake the feeling that he'll meet somebody better.

Hannah Cradick
UK

I can't help but wonder how many perfectly good things I've destroyed from caring too much. Over analyzing, over thinking, jumping to conclusions, or apologizing for nothing one too many times; or how many people I have drove away for the same reasons.

Erin Celeste
USA

One of the criteria for BPD is unstable relationships. What does this mean? For us, relationships consist of a struggle between what we feel and what we know. This internal clash can, and often does, causes external conflict. This conflict leads to us utilizing coping mechanisms like projection, splitting (black and white thinking), dissociation and more.

The underlying fear we have in any relationship is abandonment. We anxiously await it, see it when it isn't there, and overreact to it whether it's there or not.

Being highly sensitive and emotionally deep, we tend to love with everything we have. We are 100% in and expect others to be too.

We are very sensitive to the emotional changes is others. We take other's bad moods or shortness as a reflection of a fault in ourselves. This is why small slights—or perceived small slights—can cause major stresses in relationships. We want to be perfect for you.

External conflict, internal struggle, troubles regulating our emotions and maladaptive coping mechanisms often lead to a pattern of:
I love you
I hate you
I hate myself for loving you
Get out!
Not wait!
Don't go!
I love you.

Those of us experiencing BPD symptoms don't have the market cornered on unhealthy relationships! Relationships can be very tricky to navigate, even if you don't struggle with regulating your emotions. All any of us can do is strive to have the healthiest relationship we can. That is the framework I want to work with here, the relative "health" of a relationship.

I believe that it is entirely possible for someone who deals with symptoms of BPD to have a healthy relationship. I have been living in one for over 15 years.

As the partners dealing with BPD, we need to work as hard as we can to control our impulses and destructive behaviors though. It isn't easy, but it can be done. Learning as much about ourselves as we can helps.

Melanie Carrillo
USA

All it takes is one little thing, but to me it's not just one little thing!! It's a million things. It never fails, Something comes over me. I can always count on that feeling. You know, that uncontrollable and overwhelming feeling of extreme anger, sadness, loneliness, anxiety, despair and abandonment. Oh yeah, that dreadful feeling of despair and complete hopelessness. The feelings that take over your whole entire body. It incapacitates you completely. Your brain stops working. Your mind is racing, your heart is pounding, your stomach is turning, your palms are shaky and sweating, the thoughts....please PLEASE go away!! Oh but they won't. They're there no matter how many times I try and bring myself back down to earth, and before you know it your mouth is going and these things come out. Why?!?! These GOD AWFUL things.....then you're ashamed and you run...you want to shut down. You hate yourself. You hate everything about yourself. Your so ashamed.....BUT WAIT!!!!......you can't run....oh no....now you have to fix everything and everyone you broke and destroyed with your emotions, while forgetting to fix yourself. Then you sit and wonder how anyone could love and care for something so broken and messed up. So how could you possibly love yourself.

Natalie
USA

Good Night

By lying to you, I've broken your heart
I've shattered your soul, which ripped us apart
I've betrayed your love, your trust, your You
My actions showed hatred, which is far from the truth
You trusted me with all that you've got, in return what
I did was rip out your heart
I don't want you to think what we had was a lie
Actions speak louder than words, all mine did made
you cry
Your arms are still aching, from being outstretched for
so long
Reaching out to a partner whose heart done you
wrong
A promise means everything, from your heart to her
head
But once it gets broken, you feel betrayed, crushed,
misled
I don't ask for forgiveness, for what I've done was not
right
Did you mean to say Good Bye, When what
you said was Good Night

Jennifer George
USA

Ebb and Flow

Coming, going, decline, regrowth
Perceptions, deceptions; "Do I love you, or do I hate you the most?"
The pattern's recurrent
The perfect deterrent
Don't want to get too close
Just in case, just in case I end up hating you the most
But I'm scared; don't want to be alone,
Don't think it's possible to hold my own...
I pull people close, I push them away,
I'm afraid I don't know which one it will be today...
You're too close now, get away from me!
Please don't be angry, I want stable relationships; I thought you loved me
I appreciate you and what you have to say
No wait, seems I'm too angry, in fact I hate you today
I guess I just lack respect
It's not only directed at you; lacking self-respect, I hurt badly because of this aspect
And it's hard to care for people properly when I don't always care for myself
Navigating through these feelings is equivalent to navigating an asteroid belt
Idealize and devalue
Sometimes it's hard to properly show you that I care, but I really do
Coming, going, decline, regrowth
Perceptions, deceptions; "Do I love you, or do I hate you the most?"

Shawnna Hastings-Downey
Canada

Connections

My inability to feel connected to others comes from my inability to feel connected to myself, to G-d, or the collective oneness of His creation. My antadonia comes from my feelings of helplessness and outsiderness of experiencing creation.

"Why bother? I can't win." That is the running phrase of my mind. "No one will accept my attempt as valid or genuine. People, including myself, will only find my actions and words as a way to fit into the crowd. As a way to fake it till I make it."

An eternal outsider in thoughts, theology, social responsibility, and the physical world there is no place I can go to discuss my feelings. "I belong nowhere, and in belonging nowhere I belong to no one." It's a depressive statement I know, but it is no less true.

I am a dark knight walking through her dark night. In the dark even the most cunning of knights might grab a snake thinking its a rope. They might grab for their shield and find they are holding a feather pillow. In the dark nothing is what it seemed and the confusion leads to doubt and our doubt always cause division.

It is a lonely journey because it is a journey that must be undertaken alone.

Melanie Carrillo
USA

Dissolving

I can picture myself deteriorating. My skin getting thin around my bones, my legs parting on their own. I can picture myself living without gravity.
I can picture myself dealing with different, naked, strange bodies that don't care about me. No caresses, just the time for a mechanical act.
The emptiness of my self gets alternatively filled with this or that disease. I am not. I cannot. I destroy myself and I let you do whatever you want to do. Choosing is for living beings. Prove to me that I exist, and – maybe – I will live.

Meanwhile, I am forgetting you exist. I escape your hands as they strive for me. What do you want from me? I can't give you anything. Can't you see?
I give myself up to this wish for destruction. Maybe, this is the only replacement for love I know. If you truly love me, don't touch me.

Eleonora Nappi
Italy
Translated by Ombretta Di Dio

The Circle Game

My hands are wringing with an urgency to never leave this place and I sway, inhaling the terrifying sweetness of it all. The greed is leaching out of me like a stream of honey, slowly covering my skin and filling the spaces around me. I resemble something that is half human and my mind bends in preparation for the onslaught of ecstasy that comes right before that inescapable urge to destroy myself again. Tonight there is beauty in destruction, even if it's nothing more than existing in this moment without dragging up the past. As the early morning hours creep up I swerve to hit the concrete because that is the only way I know how to stop. I can no longer recall the darkness lifting. It seems to have followed me here. Was it really only a few hours ago that we lay side by side as I ran my hands along your skin? And here I am now fighting the urge to smash my open palms against your front gate. In my mind, my hands strike down upon your door and my broken blood vessels struggle in vain to repair the damage I have caused.

I'm no longer the person you knew last night. The one that rose above the noisy mob and threw my voice to the heavens. The person who smiled with conviction. The person who looked you in the eye and made you believe that everything was going to be ok. No, I am not her. I am unfaithful and unkind. My eyes are cold and unforgiving. Don't speak to me. Don't come near me with your unassuming logic. I will spit at you and grind out a spiteful word for each night I have spent alone. This is the girl that feasts upon the shadows when she knows no one is watching. I can't tell you who I am in all of this, but I can tell you that for me, these circles are hardly met with open arms, but like a moth to a flame, I dance around the edges of darkness because I secretly hope that maybe this isn't as good as it gets. That maybe there is something else..

Monique Potter
Australia

Her Pain My Fury

Tears flowing, I'm not knowing
Where's my head at, where I'm going
Thoughts are racing, fast and fury
Panic sets in, hindsight blurry
Can't take back the raging thunder, bow my head in shameless wonder
All I want it to tame the beast, it takes and takes all my inner peace
Once she loved me without pain or sorrow, I wish I could promise her a better tomorrow
I stare out into the darkness, crying tears for my Mom
Ten years seem like yesterday, I've been so lost since she's gone
I struggle fiercely within me, scream loud and cry out
At what point in time will I figure it out
I'm begging for guidance, a sign from above
Nothing heals wounds quicker, then your own Mother's love
Why can't I console her as tears flow down her soft cheek
When did I become so cold hearted, or am I just pathetically weak
Like a rabid sick animal, my words kill her soul
My actions weren't any better, I shoved her deeper down into the hole
She's longing for someone, who at some point was me
I'm right there beside her, longing for what used to be
If these walls could start talking, they'd ignite in a fiery blaze
Pain, hatred, and sadness, darkness and rage
My heart is heavy, her heart's turned to stone
We are still together, but feel completely alone
We shared laughs in the beginning, from day break to day's end
The first kiss that she gave me, I never wanted it to end
From the way that she held me, stared deep down into my soul
I knew I found true love, her heart & mine became whole
Time it's a given, Tick-tock, Tick-tock Ring
Forever my true love, what a magical thing.

Jennifer George
USA

May to December

(A poem in number about my Borderline frustration of being head over heels in love with Heather who is 27yrs younger than me.)

$22 + 0 = 22$

$49 + 0 = 49$

$22 < 49$

$49 > 22$

$49 + 22 = 0$

$49 = 0$

Explanation:

$22 + 0 = 22$ ~ Heather's age

$49 + 0 = 49$ ~ My age

$22 < 49$ ~ Heather is younger than me

$49 > 22$ ~ I am older than Heather

$49 + 22 = 0$ ~ I can never be with Heather

$49 = 0$ ~ I am meaningless without her

Kevin Harrington
USA

I love you as much as I hate me.

Jennifer Purvis
USA

When I love, I will give you all of me, and in that, I can either be a sweet dream or a glorious mindfuck.

Chloe
UK

Shards

My reflection looks cracked in the shiny metallic
a fractured nondescript visage—
human, yet not quite--
scrambled features.
Each time the demons arrive
they throw rocks—
breaking the smoothness
causing distortion.
Pieces of glass falling
to the floor–
dangerous and sharp
drawing blood.
He walks across them
time and time again–
feet oozing red
searing pain.
But he doesn't stop
doesn't hesitate to pick them up—
putting on a bandage
he walks through.

Allison Cline-Saia
USA

You were long morning drives with Ludwig Van Beethoven and Lindsay Stirling.
You were drunken awe of classical vocals.
You were inappropriate jokes at the most appropriate times.
You were hours in silence, feeling like deep conversation.
You were well kept secrets and much needed advice.
You were support and love when I needed nothing less.
You were home away from home, wherever we went.
You were my best friend, my introvert, and my family.
You were an unexplained, unspoken departure.

And now, all you are is gone... and this celebration of life feels like mourning.

I wish you were here. I wish you would be there.

That's my one birthday wish. Nothing else. Just for my best friend back.

Courtney Foal
Australia
Fighter and Survivor

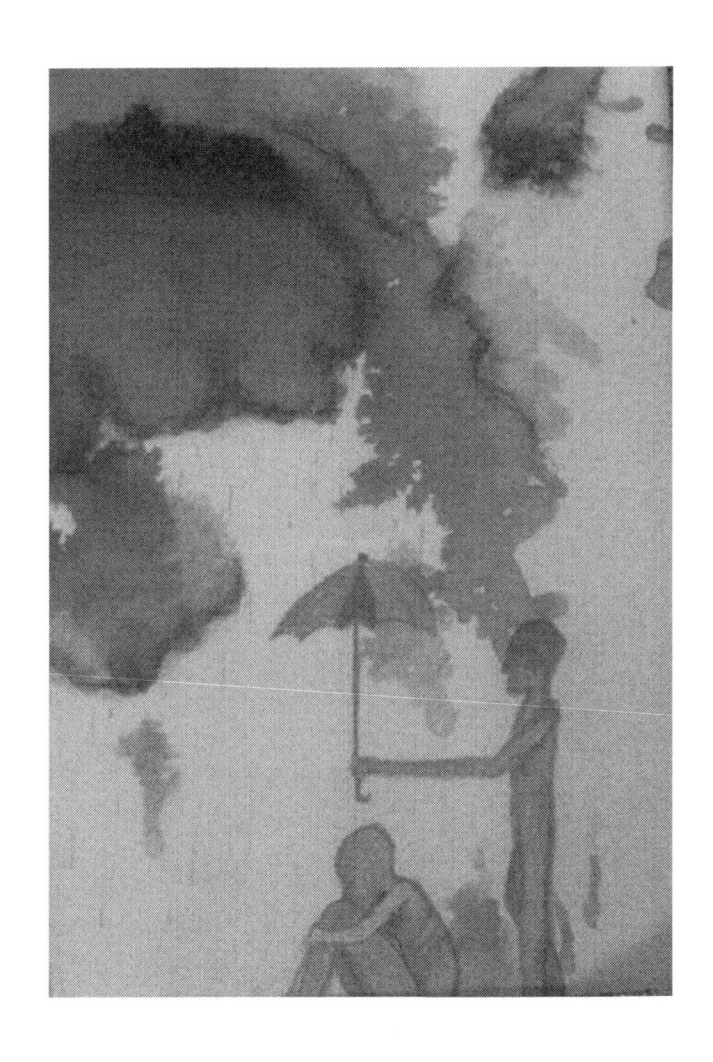

A Helping Hand

Mal Hultgren
Sweeden

what once was my everything, is not my nothing.

i never been much of a writer

but this is for someone special someone that was once the most important person in my life

but yet, i was too blind to see it at the time

i cant forgive myself for all i've done and i don't expect you to either

i look for the light but i only find the dark

i was too consumed in others thoughts

to be comfortable being myself

so i pushed you away and put up a wall

cause i was afraid of letting you in

but i didn't know it just made everything worse

we were once happy and in love now its like we never even knew each other

and the thought just tears me apart

your face is forever imprinted in my brain

and your name is stamped on my heart

you were my everything & now i'm left with nothing not even a heart

i smile so nobody can see

the hurt and broken me

i'll drown myself in sorrow

and bury myself with regrets

just to forget the hurt & broken me

-nicole bernardo
usa

Let it go

God I hate you.
I hate how you can irritate me so quickly.
How your words can cut me so deep.
I hate how you make me feel so weak and vulnerable.
I hate how you do that cute crinkle thing with your nose when I'm trying to be angry with you!

You were never strong enough to make us happen.
You gave me nothing in return.
Until you pull yourself together you'll be the same jerk you always were.
A little less of your pompous attitude would be nice!

Fuck off!
Fuck You!!
Let it go...

But that's how things always were.
Weren't they?
Laughter mixed with anger
Passion mixed with a silent aloofness.

Fire mixed with ice.

The water of our being melted to the point that we found ourselves drowning in a never ending sea of ourselves.

Now I am spinning in a small box

Questions? Answers?

Lies? Truth?

Up? Down?

I'm disoriented as hell!

But that's how it is when you live your life in emotional overdrive.

Livia Richard
USA

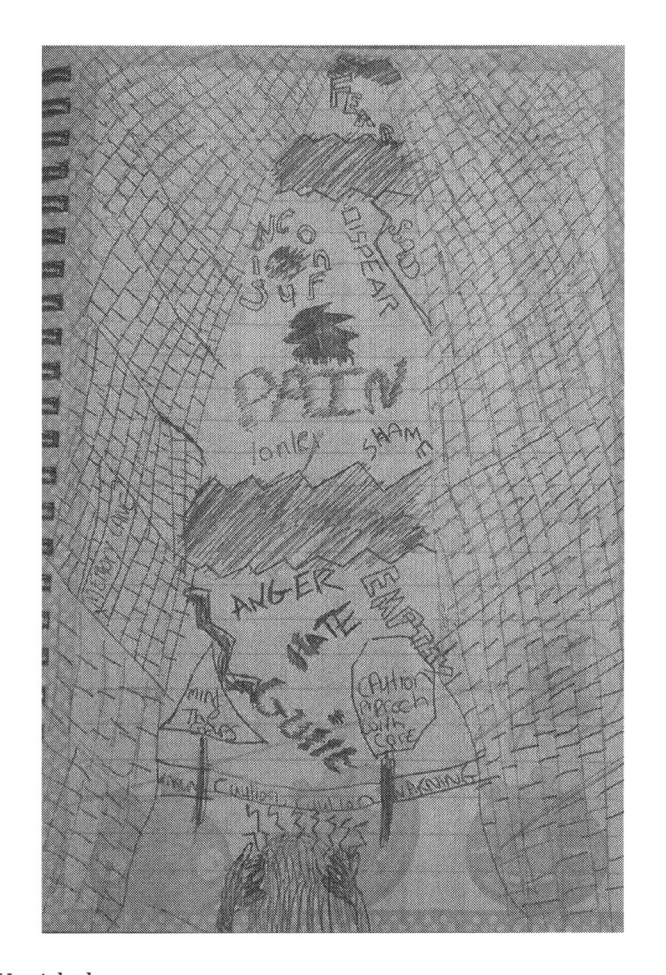

Untitled

Kirsty McCarthy
Wales

WHERE DOES LOVE GO WHEN IT DIES?

You made me feel safe.

I don't know if it was because you're built like a man, if that even makes sense.

I don't know exactly, as long as you cared for me I felt safe.

Your voice is still the sweetest sound to grace my ears. It instantly soothes me.

It's your voice. No one else has it.

But things are different.

You left.

I lived.

You returned but your love for me, if that's what it was, it didn't.

I know it's not your fault. You would love me if you could.

But your voice is still as sweet.

And I am not safe.

I want to carry on like a child and stamp my foot and cross my arms and demand to know the whereabouts of your love, if that's what it was.

I want to convince you to love me.

I want to debate the unfairness of this issue.

But you know of this already.

I want to ask you why you don't feel the way you did but I couldn't, I wouldn't. I don't want to hear an answer.

I just want to hear you voice and know that you love me and be blanketed in that feeling of comfort.

I want to bargain for your love.

But I know it's not yours to give because it left you somewhere along the line when I'm sure I was being my impossible self.

Where does love lost go?

I know you would be my everything if you could.

I wish I could take back whatever it was I said, whatever I did, but there's no turning back the clock.

I miss you. I miss the you that loved me, if that's what it was and your voice still soothes me but it's a lie because I am not safe and there's nothing that either of us can do to change that and that's not your fault.

It's just the reality of our here and now.

 Tania Neilson
 Australia

I have a constant battle with myself. Most days I am fine, except the little things I no longer care to do or just don't have the strength to do. I have found that I use love as a form of self harm and self boost. I find myself f falling deeply in love (even when I see warning signs) I love being in love… or maybe I just want to believe in someone so bad. Then when it comes to the hurt it does feel like words I read: my forest is dark, my trees are sad, and all the butterflies have broken wings. Like dying inside. Like I keep setting myself up for it. Why??? Maybe because I love feeling alive. Just to experience feelings so deeply. I hate the numbness.. feeling dead ..feeling like life is passing me by. It's a battle to stay positive, to keep trusting, to keep believing. Some days it's all too much, other days it's fine. Maybe I am sounding crazy, but these are just a drop of the things I don't just tell anyone.

Freda DuPlessis
South Africa

I react to my perceptions instead of fact. It's not you, it's me.

Jennifer Purvis
USA

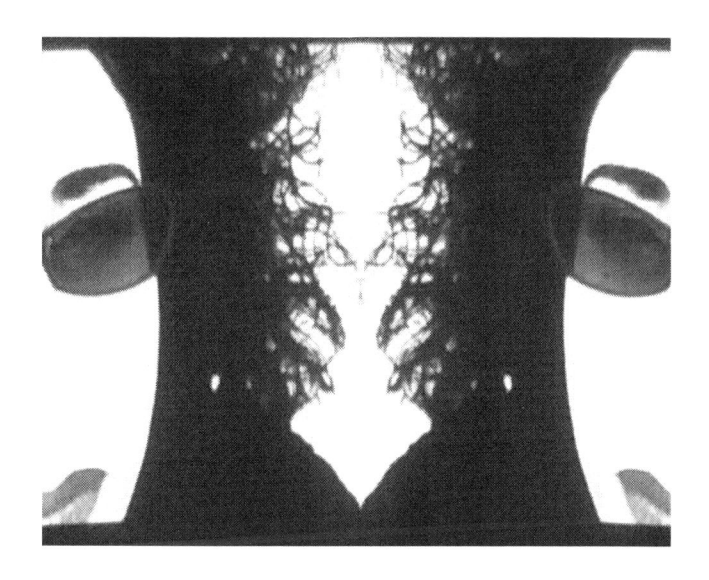

Split Mind/Split Heart

Melanie Carrillo
USA

Why did you break me?

It will be okay,
He says to me,
Yet still to blind,
To really see,

The pain beneath,
My perfect skin,
The tortured soul,
Which lies within,

They broke me down,
They fucked me up,
Then they left,
An their doors they shut,

So here I lay,
Alone and sore,
I have some love,
Yet yearn for more,

I always ask,
"What did I do?"
They always answer,
"It wasn't you"

No family or friends,
But that's okay,
I don't need anyone,
Because they never stay.

Sammy Payne
England

Borderline and relationships

Any person can be fearful in an intimate relationship. The vulnerability of being close and connected to someone can be over whelming and very difficult to process. Every human will go into a relationship with their wants and needs hoping to be met. This is a normal process of human nature. People choose to be alone, have open relationships and even have multiple partners in one sitting. For me and what I do believe every person suffering with BPD search for is the love and care they missed out on when they were younger. They long for the connection they have grown up with not having, and when the person they do believe has met their needs and it doesn't work out, it can be soul destroying for the person with BPD.

In this piece I will go over my personal experiences with the close and intimate relationships I have had with BPD, how I react when they leave and the journey I have been through to self discovery and even being able to love myself.

I grew up with a traumatic and abusive background ever since I was young. I was made to feel I had no purpose on this earth, even if my abuser was mentally ill himself. I was told I wasn't good enough from as early as three years of age, and I grew up with that as well as psychical abuse. I developed dissociative thinking patterns to help me cope with the pain that was placed on me, as at that age I was naive to the damage it was causing.

I struggled with my sexuality early teen years. I was in some what denial of who I was and what I wanted. I had people label me before I even knew myself. It was another thing I struggled with as I felt I couldn't openly be or express myself so I closed off. I closed off and didn't form any intimate or close relationships with anyone as I was fearful to be myself in this society. The knit picking of how certain people wanted me to be and to act had taken its toll on me. I became a bottler and hardly expressed how I was feeling to anyone.

I had careless sex with boys in my teenage years to 'fit in'. Noting satisfying came of my actions. It was like I was filling a void of the person I really was. I was in no way emotionally connected to these boys I had sex with. It was blank and confusing and I felt nothing. I continued to do this until I moved to Perth when I was 18 years of age.

Perth was very open sexuality wise. It was a whole new realm for someone who lived majority of her life in the country. I saw people as young as 17 openly gay and confident. It was refreshing for someone like me who was still on a journey of self discovery and self identity. I knew deep down I craved a psychical and emotional connection with a girl. I dont like to define myself with a label. I believe love is love, no matter what gender.

I had my first relationship with a girl when I was 21 years of age. She was younger and very mature. Something petrified me. For I had never let anyone into my world and I have never let anyone in enough to know about my disorder. It was a long time ago but I renumber this relationship being mainly friendship based. It was also very special to me as I was still growing myself and this person made me discover a lot of things even if she was younger.

We eventually broke up after eight months and that's when my BPD colours started to show. I was so broken but not because the relationship ended, it was because all these problems I had buried became to surface. I questioned my own self- was I the issue? Was my abuser correct in saying I am worthless? Why do I have to feel the abandonment a hundred times more then what she would be feeling?

I was in a psych ward after this break up. Looking back at the time I blamed her. I blamed her for making me feel the way I did. This wasn't her fault. It was all the emotional trauma surfacing and I really couldn't control the over bearing pain I had numbed out. I started therapy and I questioned if I ever could be in a functioning relationship? A question someone with BPD will often ponder years on end.

I had flings in between my first relationship. I met a girl who studied law and she was super lovely to me. But because I wasn't use to the love and care I ran from the situation. Something to this day I regret because I often wondered how we would of panned out and now I know what I deserve I often wish I took a chance with her. Everything is about timing and when I was in that head space I believe I would of caused more damage then good.

My second girlfriend was a life changing experience. I stopped therapy and we were together after two weeks of meeting each other. We were passionate and our relationship was purely psychical based. We had sex more then connecting. I became so use to it I thought it was normal. But something was still missing. I told her about my diagnosis of my BPD and she constantly used it against me. Made me believe I was the issue, I was the concern and I was the reason she use to lash out and hit me. I was suicidal in that relationship and I began to believe this is what I was going to put up with for the rest of my life. Days of abuse and torment just because I had a disorder. She always said nothing was wrong with her. After coming out from it, it wasn't love. I wasn't natured or treated decently even though she made me believe she loved me. I understand peoples issues but nothing can justify the pain she caused me. I was literally a punching bag and that scarred me for a long time. This relationship lasted on and off for a year. After I got out of it I didn't want to be alive. I remember I was at my house and wouldn't get up for three days. I would strangle myself with a power cord and cut myself to realise the pain inflicted on me. I tried to voice how I was feeling to her and al she replied was 'put me in your will'. Something that still makes me sick to the stomach. I believed for so long I was the issue. This wasn't the case.

After that traumatic stage of my life I met my Psychologist who changed my life in so many ways. She did DBT with me and she taught me to perceive life in a positive way when I thought I couldn't recover from it. My outlook completely changed and I started to love myself. I started to realise my disorder isn't the reason everything went wrong. We all have issues and I live the best possible way I can while trying to deal with abuse and trauma that stems from as young as three years of age. I had everything going for me.

Then I fell in love.

Now some people try tell me how I feel in this situation. I know how I feel and what was real. I met a girl last year, May 2015, who completely changed my life. I have never been so attracted or drawn to someone physically and emotionally like I am with her. I was on the right track when I met her. I was happy, care free and on the right path career wise. She was so beautiful and genuine. She also had struggles of her own she was very scared to show. I believe I have never connected with someone as emotionally as I connected with her.

The more we became close, the more my deepest issues started surfacing. I had blanked out a horrible memory and because I trusted her so much, I started to face the issue. I know it was draining for both parties involved. I was so in love I started to ignore how much I was ill because I wanted to help her. She saw every side there was to me and it was a whirl wind of a relationship. My BPD traits started surfacing the more she bought down my walls. I thought I had them up but they came crashing down. I wanted her so badly that I lost control of how I was feeling. She made me weak and I just couldn't walk away, even if it was putting my life in danger. I wanted to be with her not because I couldn't be by myself, its because I thought she understood me and she made me feel safe when we were alone.

The suicidal tendencies started coming back when issues of my came to the surface. Often the partner blames themselves if they don't understand the disorder. I do believe no one can make you feel the way you feel except for yourself. But certain things can trigger someone with BPD. Even if my ex partner wasn't aware, some action she did may of caused an emotional flash back or painful memory which would then bring up painful trauma for the person with BPD.

I am not saying she didn't treat me poorly. She did. I blame timing and issues as to why we fully couldn't be in a happy functioning relationship. To this day I still care and love her as she pushed me to the last brink which also pushed me in the right direction to continue on the path I was on.

To conclude this piece, BPD people are capable of a stable and functioning relationship. We are in no way to blame for the end of relationships or the issues of a relationship. I have read articles on the internet stating to 'never get in to a relationship with someone with BPD'. This is offensive and hurtful. BPD people are some of the most emotionally intelligent people you will ever meet in your life. Once you are educated on this disorder and realise we cannot help how we react to pain is when you will have a successful relationship. I would rather be with someone who can relate to me emotionally then a psychical based relationship. We want to live at ease and to know what love feels like. We have a lot of love to give, and its not a crime to want the sane type of love and care back.

Carissa Wright
Australia

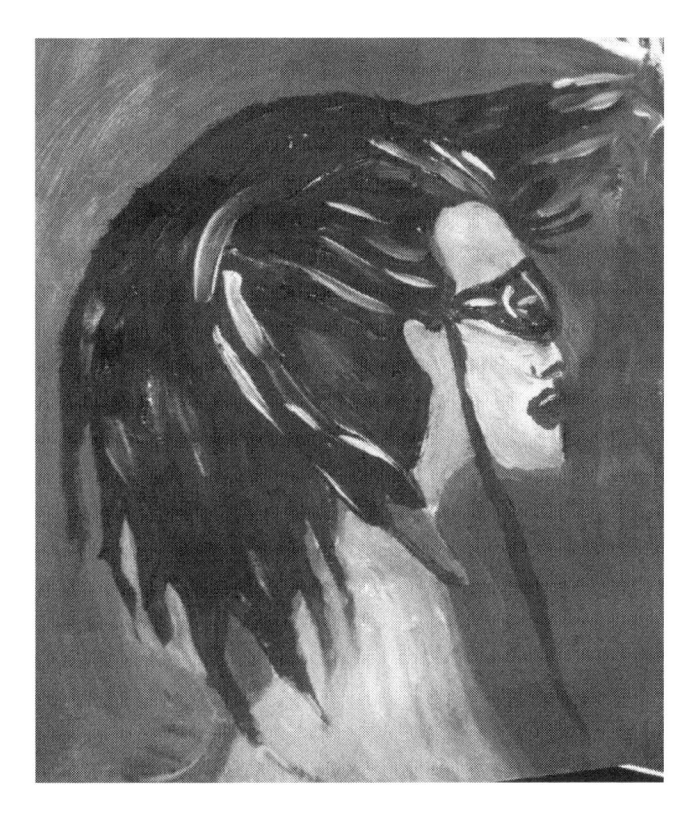

Untitled

Tee Taylor
UK

Love

How long until we get to the moment you decide to accept or reject me?
Declare or deny me?
Love or hate me?

I want to tell you I fell last night.
Hitting the floor, my heart shattered.
I don't know how to put it back together.
There are too many cracks.
Too many gaps.
Too many spaces where the cold flows through.

My inner self is freezing.
Once you were my warmth.
Now you are the ice that breaks apart my being.

Maybe that's how it's supposed to be?

Maybe I have to be broken to find the person
Who drapes me,
Filling in the void,
Who makes me appear smoother to the outside world.

Maybe I have to be broken to learn how to love?

I hope that's true.

Livia Richard
USA

WISH I WAS A VAMPIRE

I wish I was a vampire
Then my pain I could turn off
I chose to feel immensely until the bliss
returned to empty
I could end the suffering completely
Like a flick of a switch, so easy
I wish a vampire

In fact we're not dissimilar
They are dark and broody
Like me they are too moody
They romance in the melancholy
They embody shame and guilt aplenty
I wish I was a vampire

My body would mimic a goddess
My hair would be shinny and lush
My breasts would be robust
I would be slender but strong
To underestimate me would be wrong
I wish I was a vampire

For many reasons and more
But mostly for today
I wish my pain away

Tania Nicole
Australia

What is Love?

I am not sure what it means.
Is it the echo of a whisper etched onto the
invisible heart?
Or maybe it's that comforting feeling of
another soul's affection for you; regardless the
cost.
Could it be a mutual relationship built on trust,
encouragement and friendship?
Possibly Love could be the tenderness of a
hug, the empathy in an apology and the
thought behind a kiss.
No, this can't be what Love is.
Love has to be the empty apologies and
broken truths told to another.
Wavering personas fitted for a use, dependent
upon the outcome.
The lack luster treatment of words and tones
used on those you tell.
Love. Not an emotion or feeling at all. I realize
it now; Love is just an empty word. An empty
promise.
A reason to continue with hope that it still
exists.
Love. Just a pivotal, void less word.

Star Williams
USA

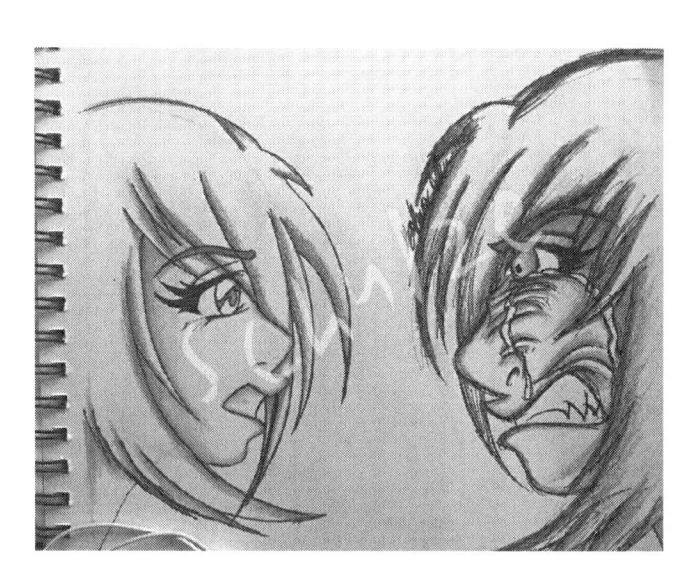

BPD Rage

Shannon Schulze
USA

I've managed to destroy myself. I'm done living a lie . . .

This journal is anything but a happiness manifesto. I hope if anybody ever reads this, they'll learn exactly how to not live their life. I've destroyed so much. All my insisting that nothing was happening with Deborah . . . It was all a lie. We were together. It continued until last month. She asked me to choose . . . I wasn't ready. I had to take a serious look at what prompted me to behave in such a way. I quickly identified the tipping point: feeling isolated in my marriage. But what was the cause? Catherine is such an amazing person. It wasn't anything she did. Not really anyway. It was me. I hated myself. I was unlovable. That is NOT Catherine's fault. Then along comes this girl . . She understands what I'm going through. She's heard the demons and knows how to quiet mine. She made me feel less alone. Suddenly I didn't have to lie about who I was. It's my fault. I should have been honest about myself with Catherine. I had fallen in love with another. Being in love with 2 people is the deepest torment I think the heart can know. I never stopped loving Catherine. Not for a single second. I loved our life together. Everything about it, save the emptiness.

By the time I was ready to choose, Deborah had had enough of me. It wasn't just the waiting. I had been truly terrible to her. In a moment of weakness and self-doubt, I actually questioned her rape. I suggested she was lying. Who does that?? I held her past against her. I dredged up past experiences without reason or fairness. I projected my insecurities into our relationship, robbing her of confidence. It was too much. She doesn't want me back.

In my misguided efforts to try and keep 2 people happy, I've ruined the happiness of 3. I

was a jealous, obsessive, unrecognizable boyfriend, and an absent husband.
I have failed. I have no hope. I have no love from either one. I am going to be homeless. I have no interest in dating or finding someone. There is no one else. Most people feel torn asunder when they lose "the one". I managed to seek out and lose 2. I am the cut that just won't stop bleeding. I am the monster. The destroyer. I breathe loathing and hatred. I burn happiness to a pile of ashes, leaving a smoldering, barren hellscape in my wake.

My demons won. I can't keep Domino at bay anymore, he wins. I'm not angry, not even with myself anymore. But there is only one way I know to stop the monster from causing more damage. You don't rehabilitate a monster, you kill it. Yes, sometimes there is some collateral damage, but it is necessary.

I'm so sorry to those I love, to those who will be affected by this. I hope you will allow yourselves to heal and find strength and love again. To my incredible wife, you were ALWAYS enough. It really is me. I know that doesn't ease the pain of betrayal, but maybe it will help you move on and find the love you deserve.
Please forgive me.

Hopefully a few things become apparent from reading this entry. I feel different people will discover different revelations in there. A couple of things that I've begun to understand from this are that A) My use of ellipses is obnoxiously over the top. B) I tend to really lay it on thick with the self hatred. It's embarrassing, really. C) This is only possible for me to understand now that I'm looking back a few short months later, but the demons return. And worse than that, they turn you on the person who once quieted those demons. The reason? They didn't actually combat your demons, they hid behind them. I guess in some ways, it is easy to blame that person, given that they appear to have helped disguise your demons while in their presence. Perhaps they are to blame. Deborah definitely had a motive in helping me feel better about myself. She understood that Catherine wasn't great at helping me feel better about myself. She's a smart person. She played on that, told me I was good at my trade, validated my feelings of isolation, and made me feel wanted in such a way that I had convinced myself that I wasn't already wanted.

Yes, my Depression, Anxiety, Type 2 Bipolarism and Borderline Personality Disorder are complete dicks. But I chose how to respond. I chose not to let happiness come from within. And now I am paying dearly for it. I hope that as I bring more light to my situation that someone will identify with these situations and seek help before they bring themselves to the same point. I had always wanted to be heard and truly empathized with. I hope someone can find that in this.

Nate Brown
USA

My Soul within Yours

Until I learn to wear the facade of happiness, and the mask of serenity, you will never consider me as a person who could have been your rock.

You expected me to be the one put together the pieces in your mind, but what you never understood is that I have never been able to put together the pieces in my own.

I tried to do the impossible.
Make you understand that you are worthy of love.

Never understanding what I wanted, you threw me off.
Never seeing I had the best of intentions, wearing my heart on my sleeve, you made me the enemy.

From the beginning I could see the end of the road but I follow it anyway, stubborn like a mule, and in the end my heart was filled with daggers.

I am not mortally wounded, but the pain inflicted upon me can be seen in my face, and I cry even though the actions have long since past.

What I've learned:

Honesty doesn't mean you have to bear your soul, it means you have to stop telling the lies that continue to injure it.

Rachel Coen
USA

(Don't leave me)

I don't care for writing
if you don't read me.
I don't enjoy playing
if you don't listen to me.
My beauty makes no sense
if you don't appreciate it.
My scent has no meaning
if you don't smell me.
I don't want to live
until you come back to me.

I can't believe you still feel like touching me, kissing me, finding pleasure in me. My body is not appealing nor seductive; my words are monotonous, my speaking is idle, my eyes are lazy, and my hands are tied. Our bones meet, but you look at me, and you smile, and you sigh, and I'm terrified of exhausting you. I'm sure I'm exhausting you. Would I try to be there more, I would unfortunately show you my real self. But my real self is not enough. I see opportunities all around me. My eyes get lost in everything and everything suddenly becomes nothing.
I never know what I want. Sure, I want to hug you, feel your skin, and then what?
You disappear. I disappear. I need to be reborn over and over. What's wrong with you, why do you keep looking for me when all you need is warmth?
Will you stop today? Will you cease once I show you what I really am?
Is this fear the reason why I can feel you so close, and then so far and, finally, not there at all?

I'm in a bubble that makes everything softer; it prevents me from being there, from feeling my anxiety. My bubble is like a pillow; the pain can't hit me.

Eleonora Nappi
Italy
Translated by Ombretta Di Dio

The One's We Let In

This afternoon it rained, and with that rain fell loneliness. And that loneliness fell on me and it seeped into my skin while I stood there and watched. I didn't move. I didn't say a word. It was almost as if the stillness would somehow save me. It didn't though. The rain wasn't washing away the sadness and tears like it does in the movies and the songs you hear on the radio. The rain was the sadness and each tear drop held what seemed to be a piece of everyone I loved. A portion of loneliness that I wanted to take away from them. My body drinks up the rain as though it has seen drought and I hold out my arm because somehow it's a comfort to watch. Like a needle etching a tattoo over my scars, it paints a picture of someone I used to know so well but who disappeared without a trace. I try to make Joni Mitchell's haunting voice take me further back. Back to a time where different faces, different minds, different hands assaulted my barely adult heart, because 'back then' doesn't hurt me anymore. I feel a twang of nostalgia for those distant memories, but mostly indifference. The indifference feels like a land declaring peace. A land that none of us will ever know. At least not in this lifetime. When you disappeared, I was left stranded in a field of live mines that I had put there myself but couldn't quite recall exactly where. Was I making myself dodge my own bullets or was I telling myself that I had once had a chance to keep things in line but messed up again? A stale pot of land mine soup that I force myself to drink. With each cold mouthful I feel the bitter lumps slide down my throat. Each mine slowly makes its way inside me, and explodes inside my stomach. My stomach becomes thin like a perforated sack, but I know it won't completely give way until I feel every last one of those bastard mines go off inside me. I punish myself for not being the person I should have been or the person you wanted me to be. I punish myself for knowing that you weren't the person I wanted you to be either but I made myself believe you were for the want of safety and a place to call home. I punish myself for the crimes that I didn't commit, but may as well have. Your eyes were often hollow and your callous demeanour frightened me, broke me, and brought me to my knees. You need not be concerned about being painted in a terrible light because I've tarred myself with the same brush. You picture me standing strong amongst my formidable army of thousands, but my army is nothing more than a hundred hollow knights mounted on horses that are already dead. They become my enemies as one by one they topple to the ground in a race to be the first ones to hear my final breath. A parting gift from you.

Monique Potter
Australia

"For You Who Do Not Know."

I live with an injury that bleeds but you cannot see blood
You see, blood is not always red
For some it is very often blue
Starved of Love and Connection
That to some of us is as valuable as the air you breathe
We were not all made the same
Some of us have experienced and felt things that have crippled us
This is not a plea for your pity
No, is it is not about taking your precious energy
We know how valuable that is
This is about making a bridge
Connecting points of view
If you care to
I hope you do
Cause we have things to learn from one another
You teach me how to move on
Life ain't so bad after all
We know this
But those of us emotionally damaged
do not always have the tools to cope
With just the simple things you do not even think twice about
Simple things ...
Getting out of bed
Eating
Brushing your teeth
Going for a walk
Talking with friends
Reaching out to Loved Ones
WOW, can you imagine that things could feel so overwhelming that dying would be easier
And that is not a cop out
That is reality for some of us
You see, inside damage is not like a broken arm or leg
It is a broken heart
Or a broken soul
Or a broken chemical pathway inside
Or a brain/hormonal disturbance
And who really knows anyway
The "experts" don't

So Please ... I implore you
Though the answer may seem simple, easy, effortless
It is not for some of us
And medicating, hospitalizing, psychological mumbo-jumbo often (But NOT ALWAYS) is not enough
Been there done that
And I know many who have as well
You and I may not appear the same but we are in the most important ways
We all bleed
We all need Love and Connection
We all need to be comforted or left alone when we grieve
We all need to feel part of something
Not alone for TOO long
Some of us, by experience, have had no choice but to be alone and try to figure it out
Perhaps TOO much
But that helps me now to share hope with you
Please do not judge and criticize
Please do not expect your core beliefs to work universally
Please time to listen and care
Someone needs you
And some are too afraid to trust and GO THERE
But it is a good moment
RIGHT NOW
And I know this moment will not last
So while my heart and emotions are still
I beg you to be Compassionate
Be kind
Be gentle
Cause we are broken
Little pieces of us are scattered all about
And maybe you can help us find them
Cause WE are worn out trying to find them
Love and Light and Keep Bright,

Nate Chambers
USA

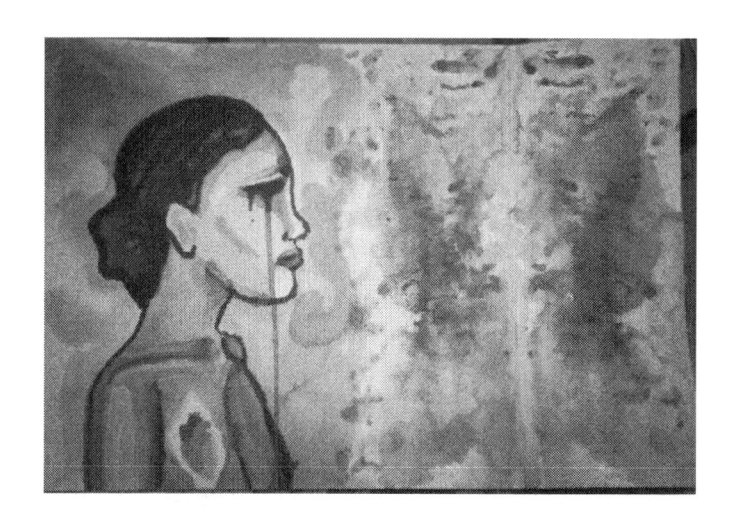

Colours In The Dark

Mal Hultgren
Sweeden

As someone who struggles to maintain a relationship with their friends, family and even parents I never thought I would find myself in a healthy relationship with my spouse. Growing up and as a young adult I would vacillate between alternately loving and hating my parents, along with everyone else in my world. No one was in my world for very long, even as a child I didn't maintain friendships more than weeks or months in length.

After age 13 I couldn't even live with either of my parents for longer than a month or so. I couldn't seem to live anywhere for long, I bounced between institutions, state homes and family members because I would either be kicked out or run away from each place within a short time. It was always after a relationship disturbance.

My first long term relationship as an adult was with a man who enjoyed messing with my mind. It was sometimes violent, always emotionally abusive and he would gaslight me (purposely do things to make me feel I was going insane, like tell me something happened that didn't or deny that something happened when it did). We fought all the time because not only didn't he care if he was upsetting me - he took joy in doing so.

I didn't even know what BPD was yet, but my BPD symptoms were out of control during this relationship and for a long time afterwards. I tried killing myself the second time while with him as a desperate attempt to escape his abuse. I was saved from the relationship by going to prison during a severe breakdown. I was gone for 2 ½ years and he had moved on by the time I got home, thankfully. We had kids together though and he would continue to torture me for years, even after I married my husband.

I am a very open book; I don't really hide much about myself so my husband knew all of my dirty little secrets before we got married. He knew I had emotional problems, he had actually heard of me before we met. We are from a very small town where he, his father and everyone else referred to me as "the crazy lady" before I met them. He also knew I was fresh out of prison by only a few months and on parole.

The beginning of our relationship was as exhilarating as any other new relationship, but there was a lot of struggles as well. The hardest thing for me to learn to deal with was someone who validated my feelings and didn't ever try to upset me on purpose. When we did have disagreements I would yell and scream but he would just calmly try to help me through the situation. Sometimes his failure to react as emotionally out of control as I did was hard for me to take. I doubted his love during these times.

Somehow, my husband just seemed to "get" me. He instinctively seemed to understand that no matter how much I raged at him that it really wasn't about him. He was able to see through all the anger and rage to the pain and hurt in my core. Occasionally my rages get to him and he will lash back at me, but it is rare. He was the first person in my life to see the "real me", the wounded child who used violence and rage to protect herself.

Without this rare ability to see beyond my behavior, I really don't think we would still be married (it will be 16 years this May). My anger and emotional instability would have been more than most other partners could have or would have put up with. Life was so chaotic back then that I am surprised that he didn't run away dozens of times over the years.

Julia Mae
USA

The Echo

"75% of marriages with somebody who is Bipolar end in divorce." Why would I wait another ten years for the other shoe to drop? What if we have kids when you quit taking your meds and going to therapy? What do we do when it happens again"?

The whole scene surrounding that question has been on repeat in my head since it was poised a week and a half ago. A scene from the same night. Standing in her living room--her living room. The living room of the house we had once happily spent our lives together in. Her entire reason for not wanting us to try and work on our marriage was boiled down to my illness and the statistics surrounding it. It wasn't a matter of if. It was when. I was no longer Catherine's husband. I was no longer Mark, the man she spent 9 years with. I was no longer the happenstance crossing of paths while she was with her family on vacation. Going to college together, enduring over a year's worth of long distance, none of that. I was a list of disorders and reasons we could never be again. Apparently it had become all my fault.

She was always the logic of the duo. To the point that I began to perceive her as cold and cynical. I had always told myself that we were yin and yang. We needed each other for balance. By the end, however, we just held each other back because of a failure to address issues. I was afraid to voice my thoughts and feelings due to the two usual outcomes: she'd either cry, or blow me off and offer no validation to what I felt. I had seen it happen far too many times. I told her how much her little jabs at my character hurt. I told her that my depression was worsening and that I needed support, but it didn't matter to her. She still doesn't understand depression. In her mind I should just snap out of it. How do you explain to someone that it doesn't work that way? You don't snap out of cancer or diabetes, do you?

If you are reading this and have a loved one who is suffering from a mental illness, you need to be made aware that you will most likely never fully understand. It isn't important to fully comprehend the illness they face in the same way that they may not understand your taste in music. What's important is that you listen. We don't need you to understand it because nobody understands it. We just need to feel less alone. It seems far too often an occurrence that when friends and family members catch wind of one's illness, the entire dynamic of their interactions change. In my experience, after revealing my struggle to the people in my life, I either get treated like I'm made of glass, or like I'm a leper. People tend to instantly forget the person they know, and replace them with a shadowy figure identified only by their disorders. I appreciate when people in my life show sensitivity to the issue, although an over compensation can be just as damaging.

In my experience, what I needed most was for people to care. I needed friends to invite me to hang out, ask how I was doing, and just show support in general. I received the opposite of that. My friends distanced themselves. None of them visited me in the hospital, and 5 months later, I am still a leper to them.

So loved ones, please don't forget that the same person you've always known is still there, unchanged and in front of you. Chances are, they've been suffering since long before you came to know them. The only difference is that now that you have an awareness of their struggle, you can be their strongest ally. That's what we all need the most.

Nate Brown
USA

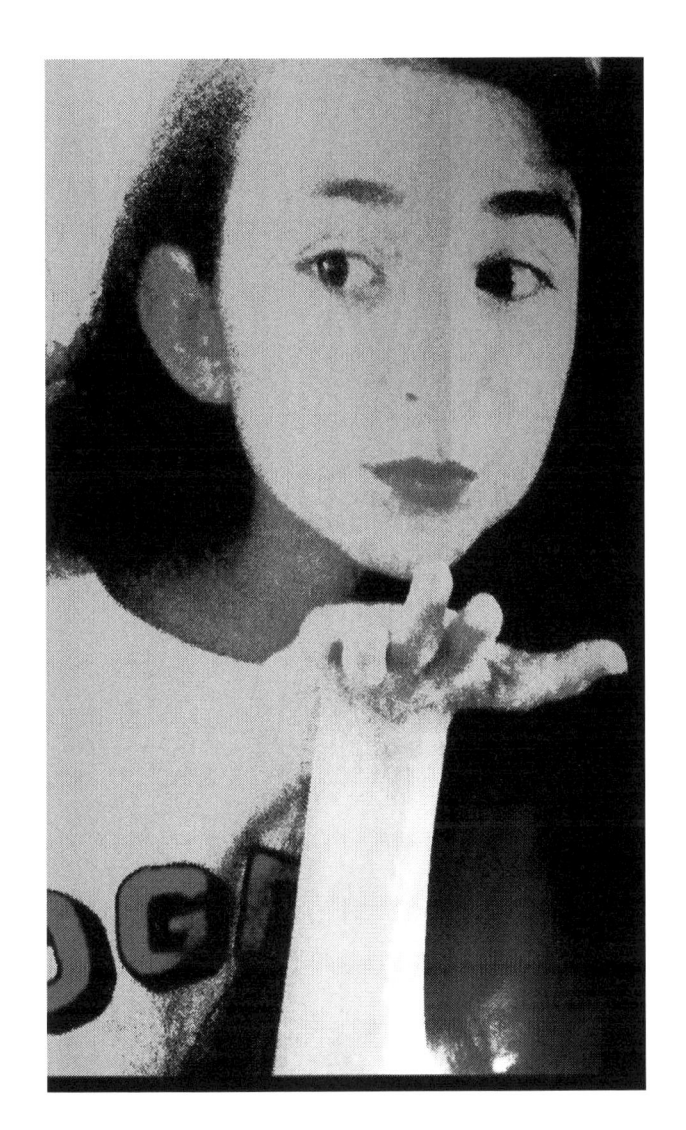

From Me To You

Melanie Carrillo
USA

III.

Suicide/ Self Harm

Today is really hard I'm not going to hurt myself (maybe cut) but not suicide, but I have this overwhelming urge to just hang myself from a tree because I feel everyone hates me.
Yet I feel so numb.
Doesn't make sense.
I'm obsessed with someone for no reason. Also I have over 100 scars on my body. Some are faded, but summer is coming soon. And I'm so scared everyone's gonna stare at me and ask questions. Even though I have a response, or I ignore them, and give them a bitch face. My throat still closes up and I panic.

I hate when people stare at me. I care big time. I've had public meltdowns and flipped out because when I'm paranoid or emotional I don't know what's going on. Feel everyone laughing at me I will start cursing and flipping in public, whether it's a stranger or loved one. Half these people responding don't have BPD they have no clue

I have a 3 yr old I hope she grows up to be nothing like me!!

Ryan Jean
USA

Shell:

I am a shell. Suicidal thoughts are back with a vengeance. I've forgotten to take my anti-depressants for 3 days I think it's been. Again I am at a point I have no idea how I got to. I ponder with disbelief how this could actually be my life. Surely I wouldn't end up somewhere like here. I would have made better choices. My morals would have led me in a different direction.

This cannot be me.
This cannot be my life.

I wouldn't have let everyone I care about down like I have in this reality. But it is my life. I have created this reality through the choices I have made.

One question plagues me; how am I supposed to go on living with this awareness? Literally how can I live with myself?

I honestly don't know, hence the thoughts of suicide. And if I were to be selfish enough to turn to someone for support, how do I justify that? The thought lingers at the back of my mind; if I killed myself my friends and family would question why I didn't come to them for help. So what is the kindest thing to do? Off myself? Or receive undeserving assistance from these people whilst causing them stress and heartache? Is that seriously being compassionate?

There's a lot to be said for the argument that they would all be better off without me. I guess I've opted mostly to grin and bear it, hold on until the overwhelming pressure has relented enough that existence is just bearable. But when is enough enough?

Now sure feels like a good time.

Tania Nielson
Australia

Inside Out

As I'm weeping
The blood is seeping
Through cuts of my own hand
A feeling I cannot expect you to understand
As the razor blade slices
I let go of my vices
I feel renewed
Emotions subdued
I watch the blood flow
And just let go...
Now I am calm, now I am tranquil
For this emotional anesthesia I am thankful
I like this feeling, and I want more
Slice again, and watch the blood pour
Sick self-punishment
Spare me your judgment
Everyone suffers, everyone hurts
Deep inside is where my pain lurks
I know that it's wrong without a doubt
Yet I still turn my suffering inside out

Shawnna Hastings-Downey
Canada

BPD Broken

People who are not in the know when it comes to self harming may see cutting as an attempt at suicide or attention seeking. For many, or for me at least, cutting has been a useful tool in which to shut out the chaotic thoughts inside my mind. For many years I have suffered with a mind of constant noise, anxiety, pressure, self torture and constant changes of emotion. Sometimes changing so fast its hard to keep up with myself, and at times horrifically slow changes where I can be stuck in a dark hole for quite some time. The things I have craved from cutting in the past, (cutting is something I have overcome but, yet still have thoughts of) are not to die but, to finally when all else fails, get a moment of quiet in such a busy mind. For just a single moment, just one minute, I focused solely on the physical pain which for me, is something much easier to cope with than a pain not myself nor others can see. The stillness and calm that moment would bring would be so welcome at such difficult times. My piece of artwork here is pretty self explanatory really using the adjectives as the cuts, showing how it would actually make me feel in that moment.

Michelle Trenaman.

(Picture Opposite)

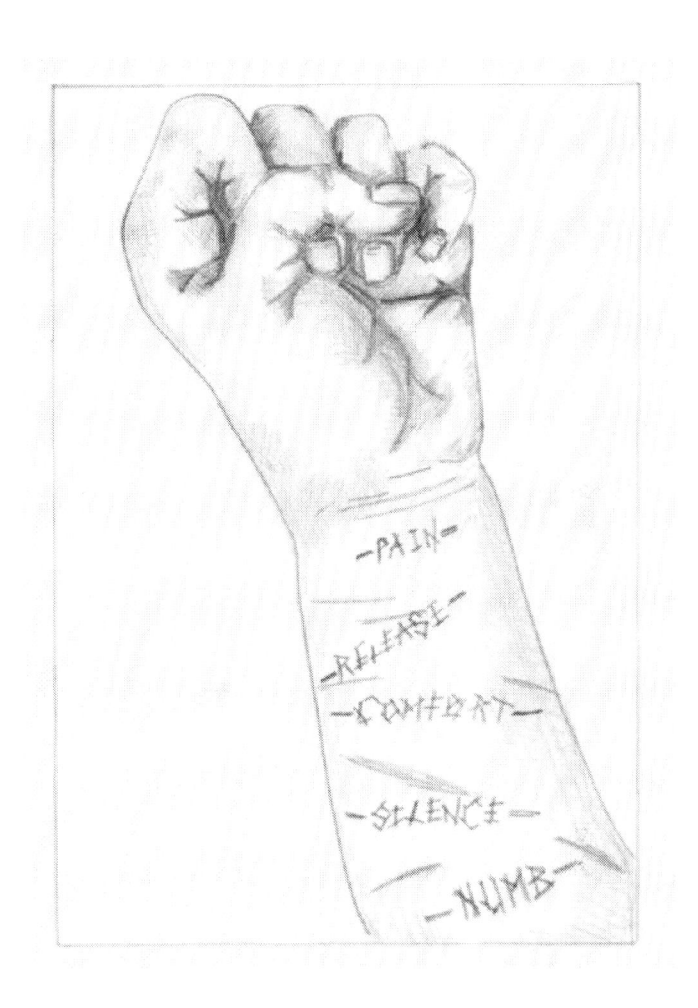

Each step feels like it's going to be the last. One wrong move and you're on your back... flat on the ice. You think we'd want this for anyone much less ourselves? No. I say to you... No! It hurts. Sometimes because we've fallen and the other times is because we cannot fall. There is this world that feels so black and white. Where is the Grey? When we can't find the Grey something has to give. What will it be? We see things differently than you. Will it be one more pill? Just one more cut? One more drink? One more hit? Something so self-destructive that it destroys because that is what you genuinely believe you deserve? To bleed out? Somehow? Physical? Mental? Emotionally? Yes those are the questions to ask. Because it doesn't matter what it is. It just has to hurt. To feel good. Former abuse is linked to BPD as well. Most of us have experienced it. As children. And some, haven't. The most common root is in the lack of validation. Competitive homes. These many things just start to spin off of each other opening Pandora's Box. You start asking... do I even deserve to be here... alive? Then you start contemplating not being here at all. These thoughts can eventually lead to suicidal thoughts. And ways... to disappear... forever. We then become ambivalent. Should I stay? Should I go? If your thoughts have gotten this far, you're in trouble. You're in limbo. How long can you stay there not knowing? Then you start asking yourself these questions on how you should go. How you do self-soothe these thoughts away when they are eating you alive? Most of us have this battle inside our heads like a war gone rogue. Every single day while trying to keep it together in the real world. We just want to break the numbness. These ruminating thoughts that won't leave us alone.

Individuals with BPD have one of the highest suicide rates. 70% who experience BPD have at least one major suicide attempt and 10% of those attempts are

successful. Some have had multiple suicide attempts and are still here to tell their stories.
Some of us are among the most intelligent. The saddest and the maddest ones are human, just like you.

Marry L. Whitaker
USA

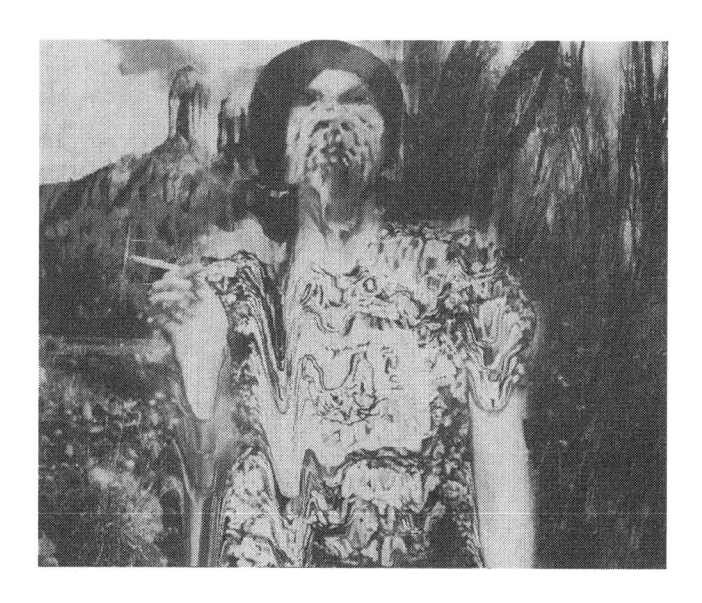

I can't tell what's real anymore

Liliana Beth Reckless
Canada

The Past That Haunts Us

Yesterday I fell, and I fell, and I fell, and I kept on falling. From night 'til morning and morning 'til night. With each breath I crumbled. I anticipated each word you wrote and I fell. You didn't acknowledge what I was really trying to say and I was sure that I was the only one who still cared. Who still hurt. I prayed to god you wouldn't be visiting me in my dreams again and I prayed you would have disappeared by morning. But when I woke up you were still there, curled around my heart.

Yesterday I missed the way you would look at me. I used to know what you were thinking by the speed of your blink. I missed the sounds and the smells of our old life and I couldn't grasp the concept of one day being your person and then the next day, a stranger trying my best to forget your name. In giving myself to you, in trying to forge a life with you, I ended up losing everything. I lost the days and the nights. The places and faces. My home. I lost it all and I walked away with empty hands and a ragged heart that was barely beating because I wasn't worth fighting for. These words are so hard to write. I don't want to write them and I don't want to make these feelings real, but here I am, writing them all the same.

I held everything in and my face smiled. I moved swiftly through conversations and I did as much as I could to appear 'normal'. Meanwhile, I felt so lonely. I felt like a shell of a human being. I felt like I was nothing. That I had nothing. That I had failed and come to a dead end. I cried silently in the bathrooms. I did my work. I kept it in. Nobody knew. I sat on my rug in Wynyard Park and remembered the promise you made to me. The promise to forever be my safe place. When the clock struck five I all but ran out of the office and stumbled into the arms of my friends. I cried and cried and cried and I felt the pain I had been holding onto all day. I felt it in my bones, my stomach, my chest, my fingertips. I ground my teeth to stop them from chattering. The chattering always comes when the pain has nowhere else to go. I squeezed myself so tightly and I cried and cried.

I haven't felt this kind of pain in quite awhile. I've had bouts of sadness and despair but this pain was different. This pain controlled me and sucked up every last breath.

This pain made my hands shake and it took every living piece of me and bled me dry. This pain made itself at home inside my shell and tried to convince me that it was here to stay, and for awhile I believed it was.

Even in the light of day, I sit here with tears welling behind my eyes and feel as though I never want to love again. Why now? What changed? Why are the dreams coming? Why do I wake up feeling as though you have just left. I can barely re-read what I have written here.

When my mind is a tornado of ecstasy and every person and everything that I see and touch becomes beautiful, I tell myself that feeling the pain is worth it just to feel what it's like to laugh and to be a whole person again. But when the pain comes like it has come now, I swear I would give anything to never feel again. I want to open my skull and scrape out the parts that let me feel. I want neither the good or the bad. I want nothing at all because right now, I don't think I can handle this pain again. Not again. Not like this. Tell me, is this really any way to live?

Last night I felt like giving up. I felt as though I'd had enough. How is it possible to feel such grief? When I'm trapped in this darkness it's impossible to remember that this feeling will pass. I can tell my self a thousand times, but they are only words. I lay here in the dark. The white pillows and sheets remind me of even darker days. This day feels equally as dark, even though in reality it can't be.

I don't know why you have come back to haunt me now. I don't know why you love me and leave me every night. I don't know why I was born to feel this way. I stare at my screen blankly. My cheeks and chest ache from pretending to laugh. All I can manage right now is to sit here and pray that this day will end. What a fool I was for thinking that I would never walk alone.

Monique Potter
Australia

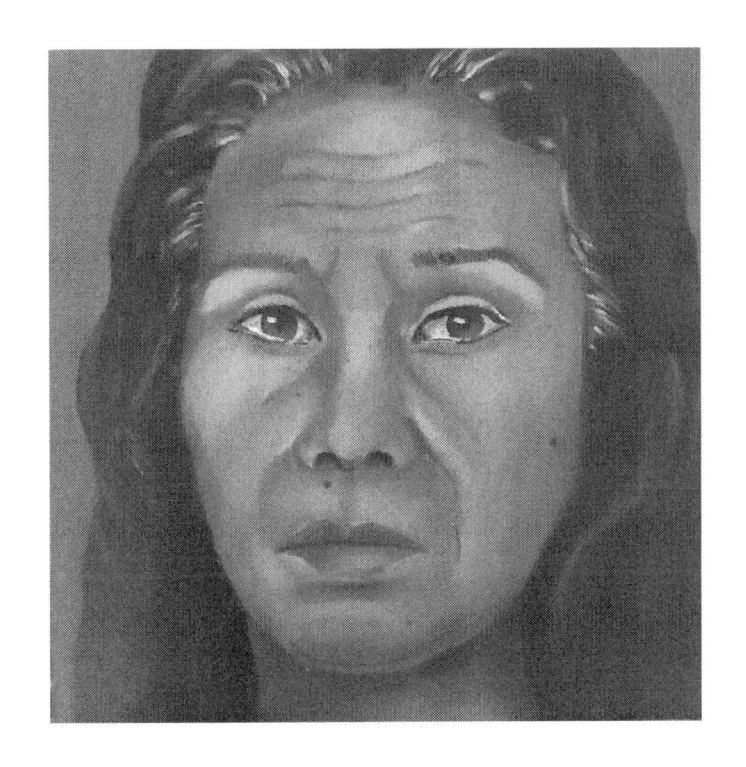

Self Portrait- Darker Days

Saadh Kent
Australia

I'm not allowed to live. Love, hugs, kisses, entwining legs, looks, smiles. They're not for me. For me is the blade sinking in the skin, for me is eating till I feel self-disgust, for me is messing up the floor with vomit, for me is denying myself life while you laugh, make love, hug, kiss, smile, say and do with someone else all you said you wanted to do with me.

Not even out of desperation I allow myself a dash to get in touch.
I prefer going back home and tearing my own skin apart, so that my body can say the words my mouth can't say.
Kiss the kisses I can't kiss.
Deprivation is once and again my daily nourishment.
I want to fall, fail.
But every gesture is paralyzed by an intrusive thought, by a stiff surface against which every intention bounces back.
My hands are tied, and I can't ask nor act.
I crumble. Upon your refusal I reinforce my image of myself: damaged, wrong, weak, not worthy of love. I take all the blame only on myself, I add this burden to the boulder. I force myself to face it. I feel the urge of tearing me apart. I listen to it.
And now I live. I take charge of my actions and of my thoughts. I'm this piece of garbage. That's just what I am. Sad, painful, plagued. I tear myself apart while other people live behind me, in spite of my pain. Life goes on behind my back, laughing at me. I don't want to laugh at myself anymore. I want to take myself seriously, no matter what it may do to me.

Eleonora Nappi
Translated by: Blandina Comenale Pinto
Italy

I'm fine,
With bleeding cuts,
I'm happy,
In my dark little rut,
I'll smile,
While wanting to die,
I'll laugh,
As a silent goodbye,
I'll fall in love,
With a silent death wish,
It's my little secret,
Not spoken until I perish,
I'll make peace,
With all the hurt inside,
The pretend and reality,
Will finally collide,
I'll accept,
My fate of despair,
Silently kibitzing with death,
So much skin I can tear,
I'll be free,
On a cliff walking the line,
They say angels can fly,
I'm fine.

Anonymous
USA

I like to burn my skin
Because it makes the darkness leave
And helps the light to dance right In

Kirsty McCarthy
Wales

I wish people understood that my abandonment/rejection fears are what make me the most suicidal, and the key to that is not only having self compassion, but also loving myself for who I am, no matter the label attached to me. I am not my disorder, I never mention it to anyone, as I see it as a way to cope with the traumas in my life, and it has kept me safe, even though it's no longer needed. I appreciate what it did for me in keeping me safe and now I seek healing for the damaging effects it's had on my life.. I also think not mentioning it to a therapist is a good idea as they get preconceived notions about how you are going to act or act out, and it's a continuum and each person is an individual. When I mentioned it to my then therapist of 4 years that I was BPD, he pretty much gave up on me and then sought to end our therapy. So good luck finding a therapist who wants to deal with it. Just my opinion, I'm sure others have had more luck.

Nancy Bearup
USA

As I lay me down:

As I drug myself to sleep
I pray I die whilst in my sleep
Please take me now before I wake
No more pain can this soul take.

Tania Nielson
Australia

My bpd started from early childhood, due to what for me were traumatic and abandonment experiences.
I am 18 now & since I was 14 I have spent my time trying to end my life and constantly hurting myself because I can't deal with the fire raging In my head.
It's sad that I have spent my years in the back of police cars, ambulances, on medical wards and high dependency units in hospitals constantly being restrained by police and security.
And still... I find so much stigma around my illness, our constant acts of self harm and suicide attempts are seen as attention seeking, when really, we're just in so much pain that we don't know what to do with it.
It's OK to struggle with bpd and don't ever listen to what other people say.
I know one amazing girl who has recovered from bpd, so there is hope and the stigma WILL stop.
Stay strong -

Candice Jerman
Australia

Yes I know every time I mark my skin
It's allowing them yet another win
Yes I know how badly it effects you too

But when the urge comes there is nothing I can do

Yes I know my scars will stay
But the pain makes the darkness go away!
Yes I feel guilty and ashamed and yes I know it's only me I have to blame.

Kirsty McCarthy
Wales

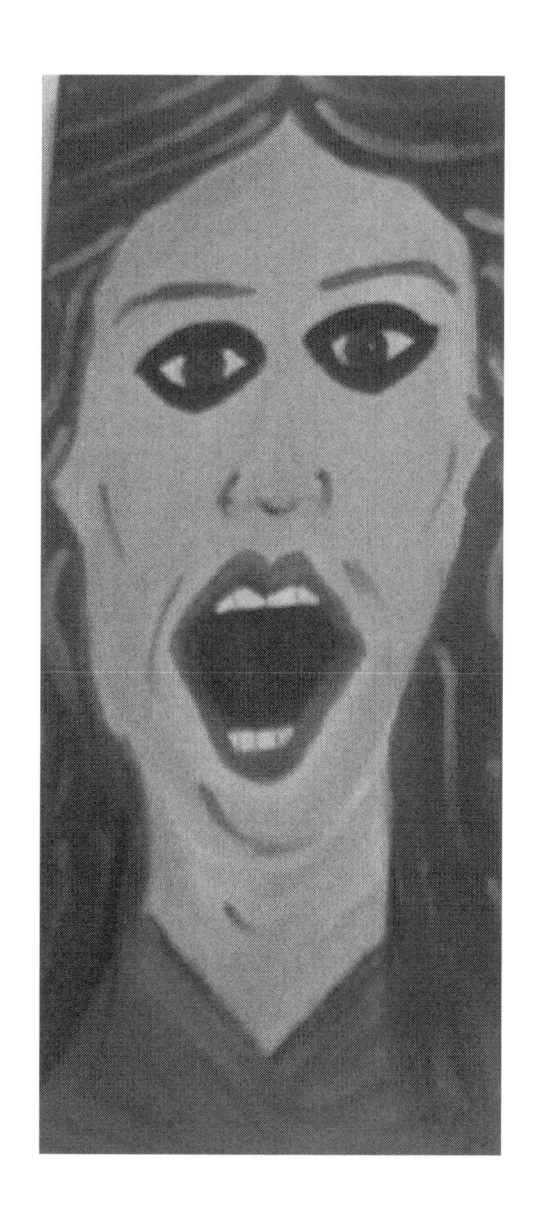

Untitled

Tee Taylor
UK

Naked

"You're the most beautiful naked woman I've ever seen. And it sums it all up, because it's when it's naked, with no make-up, no frills, that a woman's beauty can be seen".

This is what he said when, undressing me and looking at me in detail, as if I were an artwork, a note of surprise redefined the design of his face, that moved to a genuine expression of pride, mixed to gratitude and embarrassment.

He stared at my breast, saying that it was the most beautiful he had ever seen, boasting about the thousands of shapes, curves and nipples explored in his long career of lover. While I was there, armless, not sure at all about the value of what I was carrying around, and with my head down I was waiting for his response, for his judging voice evaluating me.

He lingered on my arms, touching the wounds on my left forearm, which was then full of neat and thin cuts that now are scars, memories of my familiarity with blades, punishments, life deprivations.

While he was touching lightly the rough surface of the still fresh cuts, a sad expression shaded his face, not radiant as before now, but bitter, saddened, maybe disappointed by that detail that disfigured that whole that had made him proud a moment before.

He went down on my belly, and a shiver shook me up. He lifted his eyes and saw my speechless tears going to tell him all that cut had meant. As if frightened by a menace from me, he took his hand away, but looked down at the wound and kept looking at it for some seconds. Then he bent to kiss it, as if he hadn't done anything else in his life than kissing wounds on the bellies of women out of their minds. Then he lifted his head and said: "Now I'd like to take a picture of you. I don't know if you'll ever be, again, as beautiful as I see you now. I hope that keeping this image all that I'm feeling now will be preserved too, now that I'm looking at you and thinking that nothing in the world is more beautiful than your sad eyes, than your little, well-shaped breasts, than your small but soft belly, your slender arms, your hands with long and tapered fingers, your thin, perfect legs, your slim and neglected feet."

I said yes, hoping that picture would give new life to me too, as a deforming mirror that could make me beautiful also to my own eyes.

They say pictures taken from the person that loves you are the ones that make you more beautiful, and they even say that by them you can understand when this person doesn't love you anymore.

I've never believed it, but why not try, I thought.

Eleonora Nappi
Italy
Translated by: Blandina Comenale Pinto

Suicide: An Insiders Perspective

Suicide. The word itself is stigmatized with weakness, and shame. We judge people who kill themselves as being selfish, people who just gave up. I mean really, what could be so wrong in one's life to drive you to actually end it? Yes, suicide leaves a lot of unanswered questions for the survivors...the loved ones who are left wondering why, or if they could have helped. Well I hope this perspective can help you, the non-suicidal person to take a journey in the thought process of a suicidal person, so perhaps you can better understand and either be able to help or at least cope.
I am not going to speak on behalf of all suicidal people, but this is my story. First of all, you need to be made aware that most if not all people who attempt or succeed at suicide are dealing with some sort of mental illness, sometimes diagnosed, often not. Most of us have experienced moderate to severe trauma in the early stages of our lives. Most of us were in some way victimized as children or teens or young adults. The mind is an amazing tool with its own protection method by compartmentalizing things we cannot deal with at the time. It is locked somewhere in the back of our minds, and often we think that because it is locked away, it is dealt with. Sadly, that is far from the truth. These traumatized emotions sneak back out in multiple forms, some we recognize, some we do not.
I was severely traumatized multiple times until age 14. My first suicide attempt was at age 8. Yes, I know you are thinking...how can an 8 year old know what suicide is, after all at that age children hardly comprehend death...which may be true. Perhaps I didn't understand the long term consequences of what I was doing but I knew that if you were dead you weren't here. I remember my mom always warning me when we went to my Grandma's house to stay away from all her pill bottles. "Pills will make you very sick and you could die".....a statement that immediately made sense in my small mind. So I grabbed as many pills as I could and hid them in my pockets until we got home. I don't recall the time of day or many other details, except for knowing that

these pills would make me sick or die and somehow end my pain. So, I took them all. The rest is a blur really, recollections mostly through what I was told. Turns out they were high blood pressure pills and my mom had found me as I was throwing them back up. It turned into a hospital stay and numerous outpatient therapy sessions. I felt embarrassed, ashamed and was made to feel like I was selfish and mean for doing this to my parents. Keep in mind this is the late 1970's and therapy and medications were nowhere near the standards they are today.

I had 2 other attempts in the following 15 years, obviously both failed or I would not be telling my story. Suicidal ideation is deeply inset in your mind. It can become a part of your every thought and action. We usually are self-destructive in most of our habits and relationships because we do not know any better. Our self-esteem has been crushed to the point that we self-hate, we believe we are worthless and serve no purpose. We have a sense of emptiness and loneliness that we think can never be filled. We feel vulnerable, and that no one will understand why we feel this way. We feel so insignificant and lost in this big world. We have lost the ability to hope...which is essential for survival. Imagine yourself in a dark cavern with no exit, not a ray of light shining through. How long could you stay there? That is how our minds see the world...in a form of black and white instead of colour. We are too ashamed to seek help or even mention the word because we are made to feel that way. We are made to feel insignificant. Our thoughts are so easily dismissed in many areas of the medical field. We often have to wait up to a year or more just to see a therapist, and I am telling you that from a suicidal mind, a day can seem like a year, so a year seems like eternity and therefore not a possibility. The overwhelming amount of pain that is involved to become suicidal drives us to the ideations. The negative thoughts that have been burnt into our brain, emotionally and physically for years are now habitual in how we perceive ourselves, telling us that it there simply is no purpose for us. We often have been diagnosed with some sort of mental illness, be it, depression, PTSD, Bi-Polar...the list is long on diagnoses and medications and short on preventative resources. Suicidal ideations can be common amongst these types of illnesses, but the problem lies when the door between ideation and action presents itself. Sometimes that door is opened when we relive a trauma, or have a memory from a trauma. Sometimes it is opened because our minds create it as a way to get out of the darkness. The bottom line is you can't see it, or understand it, yet we live it daily. It becomes our sense of hope, as most of us are simply looking for some way to make the pain stop. We have tried medications, or not. We have self-medicated, or not. We have seen therapists, or not. Sometimes none of that is enough to close the door that is beckoning us out of our darkness, and that is when our ideations turn into actions. It may only be a 5 minute period where our brain is so irrational that we act. We could have been planning it for days, months, or even years, and something finally cuts that last piece of rope you were holding on to. That is when you choose to let go. That being said, after 3 attempts, thousands of ideations and a few recent visits to the train tracks behind my house, I am still here fighting. Most people who end their lives are not looking to hurt other people with their actions, they are simply seeking emotional peace and see no other way to achieve it. Everyone deals with pain differently. Everyone's coping mechanisms are different. Every person has a different length of rope. Do not judge us for not knowing where to turn, or for asking for help. Instead, perhaps take a look in the mirror and try some to put yourself in that persons shoes. Try to think how awful they must have felt to have ended their lives, and question not what you could have done differently, but what you can do now. Encourage people to end the stigma of suicide. Tell them it's ok speak and ask for help. Be a voice for the ones who lost theirs, and if you can't do that, at the very least stop judging something you are ignorant about. Ignorance is not stupidity, it is the refusal to learn.

Jody Betty
Canada

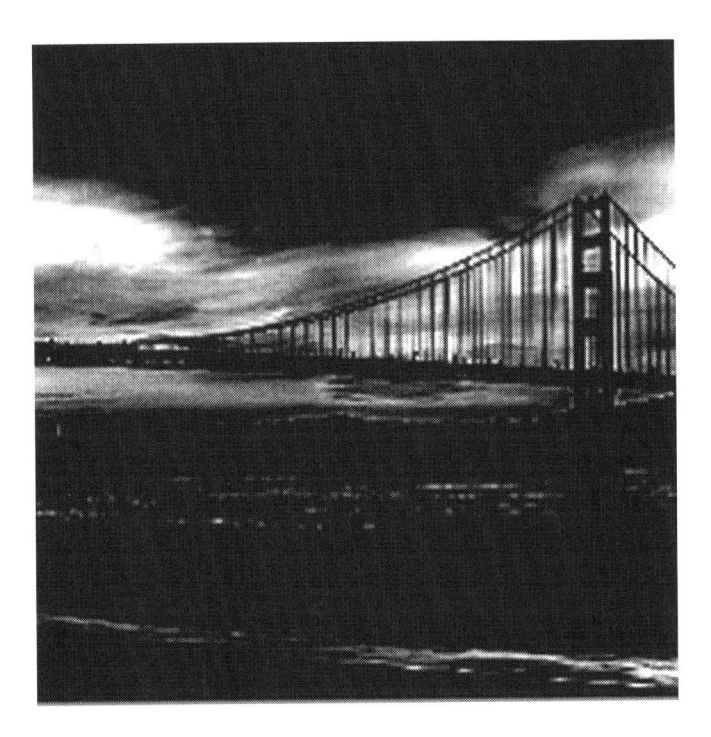

I'm a street artist from the UK.
I go by the name The Catalyst. A few years back I got diagnosed with bpd and mild bipolar. I only got diagnosed after it all kicked off with me and my partner. It got so bad I was arrested and thrown in a cell over night I lost everything that night including my partner and my son.

After being diagnosed it didn't get easier, I had so many things I needed to accomplish and prove to people, but first I had to prove them to myself. I searched Facebook for help and came across a bpd page posted a comment asking for help and a very kind women took me under her wing and helped me come to terms with my illness and even supported me by checking in everyday to see how I was doing.

Shortly after that I fell into a huge state of depression as I was fighting to see my son. It got so bad I just wanted to end it all, everyday I was making a noose and everyday my dad was cutting them up it became a vicious circle.

I was about to make my final attempt when my dad went to the shop, when all of a sudden I thought, "What am I doing? How can I be this selfish? I have a beautiful little boy that needs me."

I sat down and put Netflix on and see something called the bridge; it's basically stories of people who jumped off the Golden Gate Bridge as an attempt to end their lives.

Their was this one story about a young man named Steven who went to that bridge to end his life, he sat their crying for ages just hoping someone would notice and help. Some women handed him her phone and said can you take a picture of her so he did. He was filled with over whelming sadness that instead of seeing if he was ok she asked for a picture.

In his eyes, after that, no one cares so he lunged of the bridge, but as soon as he jumped he realised he didn't want to die, so he positioned himself and braced for impact. He hit the water with so much force he broke most of his bones in his body, as he was sinking into the depths he felt something by his feet, his first thought was omg I just survived the fall of the bridge but now I'm gunna be eaten by a shark.

Seals were swimming around beneath him keeping him afloat. He survived because of that seal and his will. He now runs a suicide helpline to help others like him. That's where the inspiration for this piece came from.

Thank you Steven, your story helped me pull through knowing you had the strength to change your life for the better and survive something not many people have!

The moral of this story is no matter how hard it gets problems are only problems, and problems always have solutions. I know it's hard at first but fight through it if not for yourself but your loved ones because they love you.

Trust me it does get easier. A year has passed, I feel happier in myself. I have my bpd under control and managed to fix things with my partner and we are stronger than ever.

The noisy demons inside my head,
They chit and chat, "Why aren't u dead?"
"Give up, give in, just do it, just Go!"
The ebb the pull, the too the fro.

I close my eyes and squeeze them tight,
I hold my breath with all my might.
I pull up my blanket and snuggle down low,
The ebb the pull, the too the fro.

The demons continue to push and shove
"you pathetic girl, repulsed of love"
"you're just a burden, broken not whole"
The ebb the pull, the too the fro.

Naomi Mercedes Broderick
England

Sometimes I think I want to die. Thinking leads to feeling. Sometimes I feel I want to die. To see only dark, to hear only silence, to feel only peace. There is something alluring about the dark place. However my children are in the light place. That is where I want to be. But you can't hide in the light. When they see me it hurts. Their judgments, their stares, their snickers, their whispers, their criticisms, their spitefulness, their need for company in their misery. It overwhelms me. My children are my safe place. They are the only ones that don't scare me. I say I want to die. But what I mean is I don't want to feel this way anymore. I need help and I'm screaming out because in reality what I really want is to live.

Jennifer Purvis
USA

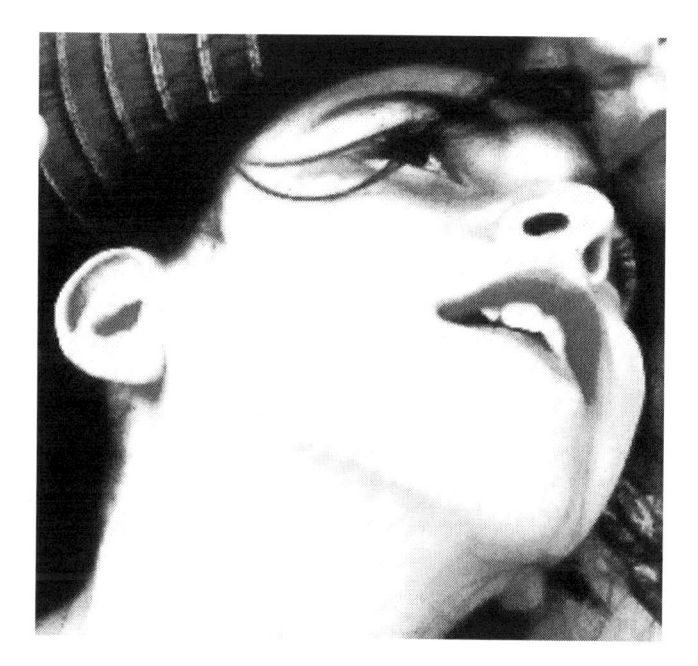

Death Becomes Her

Melanie Carrillo
USA

The Poisoned Parrot

That old familiar voice again. The one that tells me that I'm no good, that I'm destructive, that this is all there is and that it will never get better. I've given this internal voice a name and even a personality to some degree. I call him Domino, derived from a song that first helped me put a name to my self hatred. My hope was that assigning it a name would help me realize there was something to fight. I'm the type of person who after being wronged by someone, I feel a driving need to bury them as deep as I can. I must say, having a vendetta against my depression has kind of worked for me. I even got a tattoo to signify my daily struggle with it.

I've been in this place before and I've been wandering around it again this week. Truthfully, I don't ever fully leave, but every now and then I peek over the fence at a 'normal' life, and quickly turn away. In my mind, I don't deserve to live on that side of the fence. I feel this readiness to die, and the willingness to do it myself. It goes the same way almost every time: a resurgence of self loathing, overwhelming hopelessness, and no longer caring who my passing may affect. I don't find it selfish, like some less sensitive people suggest. I feel as though I'm doing them, and the rest of the world a favor. After all, what have I ever contributed to the world? So I start to prepare and wait for an opportunity to steal away and try to die. I want to go in a way that makes my body look peaceful, because in my mind I will finally be at peace, but there's also an element of superficiality to it: I don't want to look bad when I'm found. So that rules out things like hanging, guns or overdoses, which aside from the hanging aren't historically successful anyway. The very first thing I do is run out and buy all the supplies needed. Carbon Monoxide exposure is my go to method. My problem is that it is fairly easily detectable unless you can find a place that offers complete isolation . . . people tend to notice the smoke. I have considered barbiturates, but the effort needed to obtain them makes it difficult to act out on an impulse, also, even as an act of ending my perceived suffering, I don't know that I can bring myself to use a needle. It's silly, but that just weirds me out. I've also considered hanging, and have attempted to with my belt, but it is incredibly painful. You feel this overwhelming urge to swallow and the pressure on your esophagus is just not an ideal way to die. Not to mention, it is not a beautiful postmortem find.

Needless to say, I've done my share of research on successful suicide methods, and thanks to the world wide web, the information is there in abundance. One bit of advice that I took under advisement, and I feel that any other person with suicidal thoughts should practice as well is to wait to act on your thoughts for 3 days. That means giving yourself 36 straight hours of really thinking about weather or not you truly want to die. One major concern I tend to address is what if I fail? Only 1 in 25 suicide attempts is successful. What are the long term affects if you survive? There is a huge potential for dis-figuration, as well as permanent brain damage. I am very lucky to still possess my mental faculties after numerous failed attempts. Is it truly worth the risk? If you already want to die, imagine how you'll feel if your quality of life takes a plunge in the likely event that you survive.

In the moment, however, I've never cared about the potential long term consequences, because in my mind, I've failed enough to learn what I was doing wrong. In my mind, there is no possible way I will fail the next time-so I've risked it. Truthfully, I'm fairly confident I'll take that risk again, because once you crawl out on that ledge, it's difficult to swallow your pride and live another day. Usually, Domino will pipe up with something along the lines of "You never finish anything. That's what Catherine says, that's what Deborah says, and that's what your friends say. You can never make a decision and stick to it. You *have* to do it this time to prove them all wrong." It doesn't matter how flawed the logic may be, there really isn't any logic at all. There is no logic in pride.

Truthfully, if there was a trigger to this month's tank out, it was so inconsequential that I can't recognize it. I read an [article](#) on Cracked today on Borderline Personality Disorder that I think everybody should read. It brings a very insightful perspective that helped me understand how volatile this disorder can be. Sometimes understanding is of little comfort, but when nothing else in your life makes sense, you grab onto the one bit of understanding you can, and you cling to it. It may not be a life raft, in fact for me it's more like trying to float from Cuba to Miami on an old door, but it's at least a source of buoyancy.

Everyone has what they think are their limits, and they typically don't match what our true limits are. The things we tell ourselves that we can't handle are the things that we can truly manage. We need only to pull our heads out of our asses, breathe in a little fresh air and have a look around.

Nate Brown
USA

If I Dropped Off The Face Of The Earth

Would you notice?

Would you care?

Would it hit you I'm not there?

(Assuming that there is a "there")

Would you even care to care?

Kevin Harrington
USA

And she says, " how are you today?"
And I say ok
Because isn't that
what you are supposed to say
But what I really meant, when I said ok
Is that I thought of killing myself 6 times today.
That I grabbed a corkscrew and threw it at the wall,
Tore at my hair
And collapsed in the hall.
Looking at my own teeth marks on my wrist
And wonder how the hell
It came to this.

Delissa
USA

Decision

I've decided on this.
To stop my urge to overdose.
It hurts. It kills.
And I know I need to stop.
I'm going to stop.
It only kills me even more.
Every overdose. Every tablet.
Every tear that I shed
Kills me on the inside,
I'm going to live a happier life.
I'm going to move on.
I'm going to be happy.
I've stopped.
These tears I shed will be better.
Better than every overdose.
Every tablet in my mouth,
Because I'm only letting the pain out,
Not putting it on the outside.
I do want to talk about my pain.
Instead of hiding it,
I don't want to die.
I want to be happy inside
I will laugh, smile and have fun.
And forget about all this pain.
So I won't have the urge to overdose.
I get the help I need.
Through my friends,
Through the ones I trust with all my heart.

Anonymous

Have you ever been so low you considered taking your own life?
Held on with all you had to get through all those sleepless nights.
Have you lost all hope for any change
'Cause for so long you've been stuck in the rain
Colors don't seem as bright
But you promise you're alright
You think they're better off without you
And still no one has any clue
That you've made a plan to end it soon
About to leave the world - Shoot for the moon!
'Cause you've just held on for so long
And you're not feeling as strong
If they knew the hopelessness you face each day
On top of everything else, no one would dare ask you to stay
So you've made your plan & it's time to give it a try
Or just maybe you find more strength & fight to SURVIVE
Well, I hope it's the second of the two
'Cause things will change for the better I PROMISE YOU!

Ashley O'Rourke,
USA

A BPD Rollercoaster

A Loud scream comes down

Barshing trough my body..

I wake up open my eyes; got a headache ... remind myself.. Breathe

I get up light a cigarette with my black coffee. ..

Thinking to myself gotta get trough the day

I try to put on a smile at times

But the million racing thoughts make it hard each day

I can be happy in a second and I think finally a break...

But I can't get off this non stop emotional roller-coaster that's imbedded in me

I go from calm to full of anxiety. .

Oh why can't I stay still

I go from sad to angry

I try to control myself, don't hurt others

And I beg quietly to self please

Don't cut too deep TEARS down my face body full of scars
oh why can't I Stop...

And in this sadistic roller-coaster that I am trapped in with no way out of it

It goes in circles oh but when it stops

Fear builds within me as to where is it going to start at again

Going backwards so fast bringing all the painfull memories from my past

Oh how it hurts so bad..

It spins me shakes me forcefully up and down

And when the emotions are too high

From happy to sad to angry to fear

It's an explosion within me

Emptiness, I am left Numb

How can I explain to anyone what is going on when at times I'm not aware

When at times it all seems like a blurred

You look at me n think I am Fine

There I am standing tall in my high heels hair and makeup done..

You look at me and see a beautiful girl

I look in the mirror and a stranger stares back at me

It feels like being trapped in a small room in a high abandoned building

And as a cruel joke it lights up in fire

There's only one window and that's my only escape

Now the question is each time

Do I stay n feel the burning flames do I stay still n wait till the torture finally ends or do I jump out because the distance to the ground don't seem to bad and the few seconds of peace seems like freedom before I hit the ground.

Yanelis E. Rodriguez
USA

I went through a lot of trauma at a young age, and I found it hard to deal with. At a young age (7 years old) I use to lie about a lot of stuff, just to gain attention. When I was 9 years old, that was the first time I self harmed. I was fine until 12 years old, when I started struggling with mental health.

At the time, I had a best friend who I dearly cared about. She told me she had a cancer, which turned out to be a massive lie, but it broke my heart. At the same time; in was struggling with hallucinations, mood instability, flashbacks, nightmares, dissociation, anxiety/paranoia and delusions.

I started self harming all the time, threatening to take my life, attempting to take my life. Within a year, my self harm escalated, and became very severe. I was admitted to hospital all the time, was having to have stitches, I use to burn myself, and bang my head of walls. I ripped my hair out, I scratched my self, and worst of all, I broke my own wrist.

At the age of 15, I was admitted to my first psych ward, eventually under a section on the mental health act. This led to numerous lengthy psychiatric admissions. I struggled with my mental health issues. In 2012 at the age of 18, I took a massive overdose which resulted in me been in a coma fighting for my life. Luckily, I survived.

From 2013 I was taking many overdoses as well as self harming and been admitted all the time, I was very chaotic. In 2014, I got with my now fiancé. In the early months I was with him, I was overdosing, self harming etc. It was when we decided to try for a baby, and when I found out I had fatty liver disease, that I knew I needed to change. In a way, I wanted to change. And I did.

I'm doing so well. I'm still in mental health services, and I still have bad days. But that's ok. I'm happy to be out of those chaotic times, and I'm a lot happier. I wouldn't be where I am now without my fiancé

Anonymous

The pill

Why am I so furious? Nothing's happened. He said one little thing and I feel isolated in my own mind. I can't breathe. Oh god I'm loosing control. Stop! Stop! Please stop!

I can't.

Butterflies with needles at the tips of their wings flutter inside me. It hurts. Even when you touch me to calm me down feels like hot sick down my arms. Don't touch me!

These tears, flowing aggressively down my cheek burn my skin. They taste like sorrow. "It's not the end of the world." Oh god here it comes again. Like a tsunami of darkness I am consumed by my own mind again. Telling me, well of course it isn't the end of the world. It might as well be for me though when I feel the pain of my own despair.

"Just calm down" Ok. Ok. Like the straps of a backpack I'll just grip in my head calm. Here I go. Gripping and ready…….Calm. Wait. How do you calm? What's calm??? Oh no. I can't calm down. I think one of my straps broke.

Ok ok I just need to think of happy things, like the first night we ever hung out, oh that was bliss. Why did the other strap just break? I'm becoming filled with grief. I feel like I lost a loved one. I miss that night, I wish I could just go back and relive it.

What if we will never be happy like that again?!

The hopelessness is setting in. Frantically searching for anything to just make it stop! "Shannon seriously, I'm done with this." NO!!! I'M SORRY!!! Don't walk away! Don't leave me! The despair has turned into full fledged desperation.

I can't breathe.
I can't see.

It's all RED.
Where am I?

I can't find myself in this madness. My own personal insanity. Wait! I'm calming down! (That's a lie) this point calm won't break through the chains of derangement. It hurts. My eyes feel like someone has hit me in both of them. My cheeks feel over stretched as if I was laughing at something for a longer period of time. My insides feel like knots. Hard knots. I just want the anger to go away.

"Please help me!" I say "please make it stop!"

How do you fix something you can't see broken? What sort of cast do you put on a brain till whatever's broken off seals back? "Did you take your meds?" "I'm so sorry, I was so busy today that I forgot." After swallowing about 10 different things a rush of drowsiness and becoming numb instantly takes over. Like it never happened. Like it never was. The day can now go on. With no issues. As long as those meds are taken, to cast my broken brain, then all is well.

But then......who am I really? Am I really just a banshee without mercy willing to prey on anyone and anything. Or did something snap and the meds make me who I really am?

But I feel so sluggish.
So cold.
So without emotion.
Is that me?
Who am I?

Shannon Schulz
USA

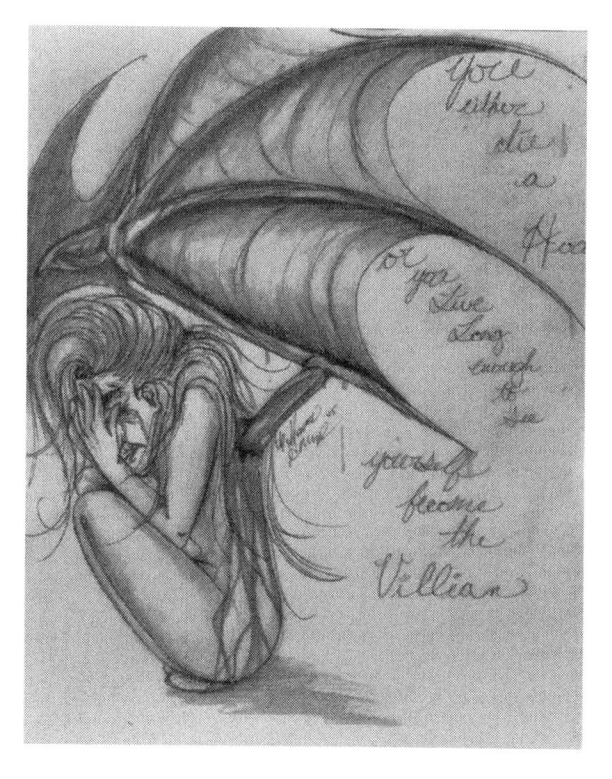

You'll either die a hero or you live long enough to see yourself become the villain.

Shannon Schulz
USA

The first time I cut myself was when I was sitting in my 7th grade classroom- my pencil box open with a geometry compass sticking out and staring loud at me. I picked it up and put my hands under the desk and scratched my skin. I breathed in deep, as I could feel the blood droplets blotting up on my skin. Since then, I'd called myself the cutter. As years passed by- my cuts were deeper and longer; my instruments more varied. I had a box of my paraphernalia in my drawer- a ball of cotton (for aftercare), mild sedatives and sharp objects.

I think I'd loved blood since the time my mother stabbed a pen into my arm. She looked at me regretfully after minutes of noticing the blood, while I stared at it with amusement. I loved the little spherical pool glowing ruby red. I had fallen in love with how the vast amounts of suppressed emotions purged through my skin as the river rolled down like tears. I'd always cut in areas that were normally covered till one day- I decided to show the world who I am. Broken and fragmented. So I took the knife and cut parallel lines into my skin. And when it was over and there was a pool madly rushing out, I realised what I had done to myself. I'd left my scars open for the world to see how crazy I am. And the Gods above punished me more for not treating my body as a temple and I developed hypertrophy. My scars blazed for everyone to see and notice me, and I wore long sleeved shirts even in the heat of Indian summers.

Till one day the light passed through my cracks.

It was one afternoon when I was sitting in my hostel room after a therapy session of inner child healing. The joint lit between my lips, I could see the pieces of me stringed together. It wasn't me. I wasn't the crazy one. My environment was. I'd been abused since I was five years old- physically and emotionally. Most of my attempts at self harm had been out of anger for another human being and a mild bump that could drive my vehicle off the cliff named suicide.

I started finding myself again. I found myself in the music that I listened to and created, getting away from the toxic environment and letting go of years of conditioning. The cycles if trauma repeated till I learnt my lessons and I was ready to let go finally, see the bigger picture to own my future. I was a warrior and I always will be. And nobody gets out of the battlefield without a few nasty bruises.

Although I've been personally working with DBT- as a psychologist I have a lot to say about BPD especially as it's also one of my most favourite disorders. I don't think BPD is really understood. I think a lot of people with this diagnosis are actually Empaths with an overactive or completely blocked heart chakra. This clearly explains the higher suicide rate amongst individuals affected with borderline personality disorder. I believe that the hypersensitivity related to BPD could stem from the abusive past and the maladaptive attachment styles that individuals learn to form with their earliest caregivers that are repeated again and again like repetition compulsion. The complex PTSD is a common element with many suffering from BPD and needs to be healed spiritually. Grounding through nature, forming ties with people who are positive and supportive, and following dreams goes a long way to tear down the shades of negativity dabbed into the lives of individuals.

I think it's also important to address obsessions and compulsions related to BPD. I have wondered sometimes if I'm an addict. But all I know for now that is that like an addict- I really wanted to escape pain. I'd taken all then roads- drugs, sex, eating disorders, dysfunctional relationships which are all grouped under self destructive behaviors. My inability to comprehend reality as the dark dysphoric patchwork of grey that I was living in made me anxious addressed and depressed addressed and I just wanted to forget. Forget my sorrows. Forget how I'd been hurt. Forget how I'd been neglected. Forget how I'd been abused. Forget how I thought of myself as worthless and helpless. So I took to slow silent means of self annihilation. It didn't make me happy or provide me with an euphoria- my obsessions and compulsions helped me survive.

But I knew that I really had to love myself. And that nothing would change till I really did. I'd fallen for men who were emotionally distant or abusive, and I'd rejected the ones who saw the light in me. But my love was in hues of darker pastels because the stars didn't shine through the dense clouds of self doubt and self condemnation. So I lifted my hands, took a deep breath and held myself close every morning before I woke up. I told myself that I completely love and accept myself. I reminded myself that it was time to grow up and stop having sharp objects as my best friends, and I turned to nature. And trust me- it helped. So much.

I walk in the sun, basking in the golden glory I put aside my fears and truly live for the moment.

Here and now. That is the magic phrase. I remind myself of how everything is transient and I just want to be happy and let go of anything that vibrates lower. I've found deep love in my heart for myself. And after all these years- the fragmented versions of me have been stitched together. There are times when I feel like I don't belong here, but I know that I have come here for a special purpose. I'm made for the stars, and I'm made of the stars and nothing else. The medical community that had once diagnosed me as BPD didn't see my shine. They didn't realize that when I look at them- I can see through them. They didn't know that my emotions swing not because of my affect instability but because I can sense your emotions, and my heart was too empathetic to not feed the compassion. They didn't know that they'd have been diagnosed too or worse, probably had a psychotic breakdown if they'd stayed in the same environment.

Personality disorders are pervasive long standing disorders born mainly from nurturing problems. How is it then that the prognosis of BPD gets better after 25-30 years of the individuals? I'll tell you.

The heart learns with the soul.

I'm a teacher now. And I'd like to believe I'm a great teacher. My children have a fine balance of love and respect for me. I have finally learnt to deal with people I don't vibe with from a different approach, and I've learnt that we find ourselves sooner when we believe on ourselves and the grand scheme of this universe.

Arundhati Chaudhuri
Banglore India

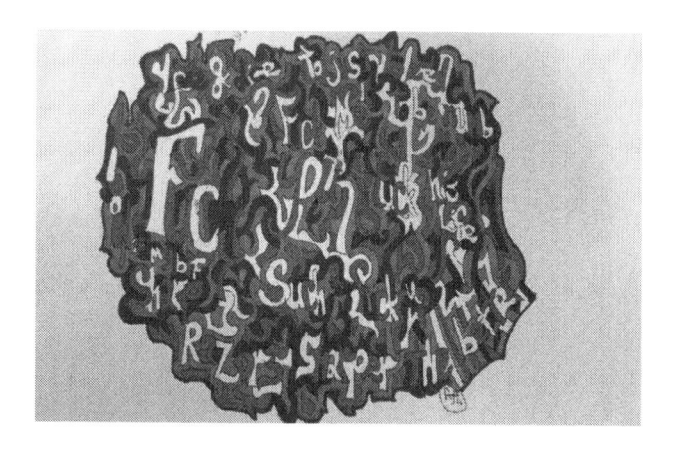

The MeAze Art

Amy J. Iverson
USA

IV.

Effects Of Abuse

I will never forget what either of my parents have done, nor will I ever forgive them.
They have stolen from me many things, including innocence, childhood, and most definitely identity,.

My Mother and her family have always lived by a simple motto - "you fuck me over once, you're dead to me".

How many times has my family fucked me over? Realistically, hundreds.

Some may say that I have grown into a very bitter man, but who wouldn't have?
Forget about all those American stories about abuse survivors who find Jesus throughout their middle years and turn into inspirational people - that doesn't apply to me at all, I was damaged from the start and I became even more damaged as I grew up.

Forgetting what my family have done to me, and how they have behaved will never happen.

I have tried every fucking religion in the book throughout the years, even prayed to god silently while my father abused me roughly from behind.

Nothing happened. Nothing ever fucking happened.

I've drunk my sorrows away, and tried to find answers at the bottom of the bottle.
There were never any there.

I've been through over nine years of counseling, only to find that talking about this shit does not help.

I've stuck a needle in my arm with a syringe full of incredibly strong black tar heroin, trying to reduce myself into a drug fueled haze so that I can just have a moment's peace without having to remember everything.

It is quite obvious that none of these things have worked, if they had I'd be cured! I would not be writing this book now, I would be living a perfect life and existence somewhere on a beautiful tropical island, reaping the rewards for my writing.

Lets snap the fuck back to reality now, this is how things are

I have been sexually molested repeatedly by my father.

My mother enjoyed the fact that I was being sexually abused by him, it took some of the pressure off her having to fuck him all the time.

My brother (my only sibling) was not supportive when we were kids, he would tease and ridicule me for his own sick enjoyment.

My father's family - we were never "allowed" to get to know them, Mum kept us clearly away from them.

I met my grandmother on my father's side a handful of times, and my grandfather the same.

They were strangers to us growing up, and nobody really saw it as unusual that we had no contact with them.

My Mother's family we had a lot of contact with throughout the years as kids, especially my Grandmother and her husband Clive (not my paternal Grandfather).

Also present throughout our childhood were my mother's numerous brothers and only sister, Lee.

In some ways, perhaps I have really become that bitter man, holding onto my hatred and anger for over 37 years, and never letting people into my life for fear of them destroying me even further.

I often think about what my life would have been like, had my father not started to fucking abuse me every night.

Surely, it would have been a much more well rounded and satisfactory existence, right?

The demons in my heard are like cancer - they're eating away at every part of me that makes me human, sucking it dry and feeding from it like a leech.

I hate these memories for that, but I cannot do anything to prevent them. How the fuck do you stop remembering?

Perhaps the act of stopping to remember is not how it is done at all? Is there a way to still remember without it hurting?

Is there some strange ritualistic dance I can perform to rid myself of these demons and feel normal, perhaps?

Fuck, throughout my live I've tried every religion known to man - I've been a Christian, a Catholic, a Satanist, a Pagan...

I even had my own fucking religion full of strange beliefs years ago, because I was seeking a way out.

I never found it.

I never found it because it does not exist. Every time I tried looking for a way out, I could still feel my father pumping his filth into me, my brother taunting me, and my mother screaming at me, and flogging me.

There was no way out of this, and there was no way around it either.

Sure, hundreds of "easy fixes", but nothing permanent , nothing that got rid of it forever and made me feel normal and complete and sane.

I question myself every day - what the fuck did I do wrong to deserve this?

This started when I was only 3 years old, what could I have possibly done that was so bad?

If I had done chores, if I had tried harder to be a good boy, if I had not spoken back, if I had just shut my dirty little fucking mouth UP!

There have never been mirrors allowed in my house. I cannot stand to look into them, because I fucking hate the man who looks back at me.

He is a stranger. He is an unwanted entity, he is a fucking abomination of all things that I despise.

I have not owned a mirror in all of my adult life.

I've learned to cope without one, shaving without a mirror, brushing my hair and teeth without a mirror.

What the fuck do I care what anyone else thinks now. I have already left the building. I am no longer existing in my own mind.

My mother loved to hold me in front of a mirror and taunt me, telling me that I was hideous, that she wished I'd been normal, and that I was her worst nightmare. I came to believe it, I still do.
She certainly made her impact on me.

I cannot look at men, I have never been able to. I despise men, I wish I was not one. When I was younger, I begged my brother to castrate me with a pair of rusty kitchen scissors, he agreed, and we almost went through it - but he backed out when I became enraged and yelled at him to "DO IT!".

I wish he had.

I have sunk so low into myself that I have consumed my own soul, swallowed it whole and buried it deep.

There is no soul in a person like me. I have done everything I can do to remove it.

My identity was stolen from me by my parents - there were no photographs of me around them, they were kept locked in a cupboard, only my brother's pictures were ever on display.

My medical documents and passports were always kept hidden away from me, as though I didn't exist.

They wanted me to feel like I was not alive.

I am a ghost, I am a walking fucking nightmare.

My head is so haunted that I cannot wake up, and the nightmare continues wherever I go.

Dark shadows follow me continuously, the looming dark shadows of my past, forever stalking at my hells like a rabid dog.

My insides squirm with the thought of it, my head reels and my tongue feels numb.

After all of this - why do I still hope? Why do I even continue to proceed with a life that I cannot bare to be involved in?

I do not know the answers to any of these questions, but even less that one.

This is MY BPD.

I am without help, and without support - could you do this alone?

Do you dare?

Scott H.
Australia

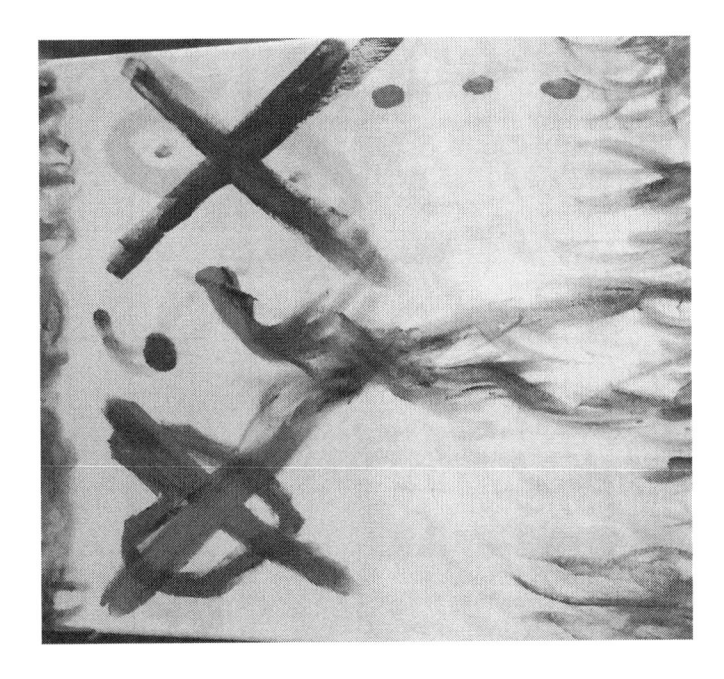

Cross Out

Keriann McDonnall
Wales

My Story:

Right now, I'm correcting OLD Loretta and discovering who I really am as a whole person. That is why I'm sharing this to all:

When I was young about 4 -6 years old I'm not sure EXACT age- my mother took me to a Women's Abusive center for battered wives back then because my dad was an alcoholic and wasn't always a nice person. So, I remember my mother being in someone's car back then I have a vague memory on the day she took me and I saw my dad turn onto the street we lived on at that time and then we left and went to the shelter.

While there at nights my mother went to meetings (she told me later in my adults years), and I was sleeping where all the kids were. We all shared rooms with other people. So, what happened to me was I was approached by 2 black kids, one boy and one girl, and they made me go into the bathroom with them and made me strip my clothes off. No real sex happened, but it was the act of laying down with these people laying naked which I didn't want to do.

I had ANOTHER separate incident happen at the same place where a bunch a girls were in the bathroom standing all around another black person, this time a boy....all the girls were white...so note that. The ring leader of this mess wanted me, or anyone, to play with this little boy's dick...no one else would...she was, and so I'm the only one felt it was my duty to...or felt that I HAD to...because, since I already experienced prior incident, and I think because I just wanted to belong, that's why I think I did it. Which NOW I personally HATE when I have to do anything....NOW I fight anyone who f**king makes me do anything!!!

Going on...

Back then, I didn't tell my mother right away what happened to me. We eventually did leave and went back to my dad because he swore he would change and give up alcohol on which he did and cigarettes...I also did tell her eventually what happened at that shelter.

I wasn't sexually abused, but my first introduction to sex was an early one and I learned about positions and boy's anatomy at a very young age in sexual way. At age 6 or 7, is when I had my first kiss with a boy in 1st grade and I already knew about the F word and other sexual stuff at a young age.

When I was young my parents went to Cleveland Ohio, and we lived there for awhile. I personally didn't like it there because the 1st day of school a black OLDER kid (I was in 1st grade.. They were much much bigger than I was...looked like 6 graders to me) put a garbage can over my head.

I have to admit something, at that time, being victimize by black people in my early days, I didn't like them...my mother told me not to HATE them. It's not everyone who is at fault. She's right! So, I only HATE those who PERSONALLY HURT me in my life....where I feel VICTIMIZED, where I feel I couldn't fight, and I felt helpless and dumb because I let them do these things to me....so I'm so F**KING ANGRY....now!!!

Also, during this time, we moved back to Pennsylvania after Cleveland. I attended First Grade at East Allegheny schools. I had no prior learning skills...I didn't know my ABC'S or what 1 + 1 was. I remember my teacher YELLING at me in front of everyone asking me? What is 1 + 1? She didn't know the HELL I went thru prior, and because no one ever taught me anything is WHY I didn't know, and eventually placed in a LEARNING DISABILITY class.

Even though I was not diagnosed with ADD or ADHD, I had trouble focusing back then. I'm glad they didn't recognize it because I wouldn't want to be on Ritalin. That teacher still to this day, pisses me off!! I admit she made me cry and it made me feel even more isolated, and everyday I suffered with fear and anxiety going to school.

As an only child, I had low self-esteem about myself and I hated myself. When a boy I had a crush on down the street told me that my cousin was prettier than me it shattered me!!! Even now!!! Makes me feel so UGLY inside. Makes me crawl up inside, and makes me want to die...

I hated myself....but instead of killing myself...I slowly began to eat and isolate, and wasn't allowed to go out with anyone and hang out with people with my own age. My parents were strict because my dad has FEARS too, I didn't know this then...so that's why I NEVER really was social....still not today!!

When I started to get fat. People didn't like me anyway...they made fun of me, and back then I didn't fight people...I had NO BACK BONE. That's because I hated myself so much I felt everything said about me was ALL true so why fight them on what they were saying about me. I was FAT this was true.....so I didn't love myself and I let OTHERS take advantage over me...

A kid in high school, a boy who I absolutely loved by the way back then, he looked hot to me, he mistreated me, used me, and left like all boys do. So, it left me unfinished...but I learned how to give a blow job for the first time. I also got into trouble back then for that...got suspended for 10 days and so did he...all because I told my cousin who had to tell her mother who told my dad...who told their therapist and he said to tell the principle and so that is how my ass got into trouble...which I had to go to a therapist for a first time, see a PCP, and other shit before going back to school again and when I came back to school...I was made fun of and he got a pat on the back of course. I hate when people do that.

He ended up moving on...literally. I did too...to more assholes and more assholes...I didn't select well in the men department because I was overweight. When you're an overweight person your selections are not many to choose from and the people you do usually get are not usually nice. I didn't know that going in.

In the very beginning I was very INNOCENT and very naive in my ways of thinking with boys in general. I believed right away if they told me I was pretty... other words I was a sucker and I was easily fooled by men who were not nice people. I was always told to wait and someday my handsome guy will come..I'm a go and get him kind of girl...he's taking to long. lol So, that is how I ended with jerks.

Before I got married I was in a relationship that I literally tried to block out because it was very very painful for me...the end result was he moved away to get away from me...and he didn't give me his phone number and that literally hurt... I really wanted to die. I was really stuffing down that food then. I hated myself so much.

That's when I ran into my ex-husband at a grocery store. We dated and hanged for a year until we got married, and after we got married that's when he told me ..NO MORE SEX NOW!!

I said, "What?" That's what his parents do ...so that's another thing he learned and passed down to me. Everything his dad did to his mother he tried to do it to me. I wouldn't allow it, but, he is very forceful and very stubborn when he wants to be. It's true. When he doesn't want to do something he won't. He will literally have me do it because he expects me to do everything for them...hand everything over to them....like he is privileged. I'm not being mean, I'm being honest.
Again, I was the one who tried in our relationship where he didn't try to love me. Granted, I wasn't sexy then at 376lb, and I had a gastric bypass which I already wrote about...several times...I literally went thru hell recovering thru that, and I also endured a lot of shit during this time with my ex-husband and his family. My ex-husband would yell at me, to GET UP!! If I could I would.

My ex-husband at the time wanted to go out with other people, his so called friends. Get this... I had tickets to see a Scooby Doo play, because that's my favorite cartoon character and my ex wanted to take his ex-lover Renee to this play!! My ex went to a special school where they still had a prom to go too. His mother said, "Why shouldn't he have any fun because you can't?" Well, Hello, I'm his wife and I had MAJOR SURGERY, he outta care for me vs going OUT with his friends at this dance.

This is why I feel hated towards these people at times...well, again, I feel victimized by them and I personally feel they NEVER helped me only belittle me and I felt I was being nice by giving them the house. I never wanted their precious MONEY. It was NEVER about money for me. I'm about LOVE & RESPECT and finding one person who shares that in common with me. He doesn't have to be YOUNG, RICH, or HANDSOME.

I personally feel that my boyfriend now is everything I've ever wanted. I really do!! Now, we are totally opposites of one another in about everything. So we always argue about everything. But, my current man, loves me and when we are not fighting, because we do daily, he is just there for me and comforts me and when I'm triggered and he reminds me he loves me and that's exactly what I need from him during that time. I can't always deal with seeing other women on TV, during naked and sexual scenes because I had to sit there and listen to my old boyfriend after my ex-husband ranting and raving about these women to me. My story is going to explain about this person.

My current boyfriend now appreciates me and does not cheat on me. I finally have a good man. So I am a HAPPY women now.

But, also I am a very very ANGRY women because after being with the ex-husband I went to another person that was way worse than my ex-husband was...this one was a little physical with me, mostly verbal, controlling, and wouldn't allow me to voice my opinions or expressions. I had to suppress my anger and wasn't allowed to show it. He would tell me all bout his PAST women relationships in GRAPHIC detail so I could get the blow by blow, and I had to sit there and hear him rave about it over and over and over again...he wouldn't stop...this happened a lot...he knew it bothered me...he didn't care. So, when I finally got away from this asshole...this is when I started to pick me up slowly and work on myself...but, I didn't really start to heal until started to walk and lose my weight and feel stronger about myself.

Believe me...looking into a mirror is reality and this helps with people with low self esteem as a way to self build yourself up. I use this as a tool to see me for me. I still have a lot of issues and I am NOT cured of my problems, but everyday I'm trying my best to get better about myself and make improvements.

There are somethings I don't have a handle on yet, such as my EXPLOSIVE ANGER. These are TRIGGERS that pop out of me and I really do try to CONTROL them, but it's hard because I have a lot of suppress anger built inside me. A lot of people say LET GO!!! That's very hard for me because I'm fighting back now....and I feel they ALL should pay for hurting me for breaking me....making me feel weak... Now I'm not weak and I'm stronger than ever....I'm not a f**king victim anymore!!!

That's why I feel the way I do. Maybe my approaches are wrong and childish, and I do admit maybe I don't handle situations right..that's because of this ANGER.

I work thru these things myself and handle these without a therapist. I HAD one, but she's NO HELP!!! We don't connect well...we are in two different places so I don't see where she is and she don't see where I am. So, I handle most problems myself and by walking. I don't have many friends or hang out with people because of how people treated me all my life...why should I want to friends with people...I rather be friends with an animal because I know that animal won't hurt me unless it would bite me...even then ..it's still not trying to actually hurt me....vs a person who is plain ass mean. I'm currently trying to have an open mind about people, but my guard is ALWAYS up!!

So, now, I feel that each person who has broken me deserves to feel what I felt, and I don't have pity on those who hurt me, and I don't f**king care about their feelings or needs because they NEVER cared about me when I was their victim. Tic for tact I say!! Everything said here is based upon my opinions about what happened in my lifetime.

Right now, I'm discovery mode and learning ALL that I can. That is why I am adding myself into various groups. Since really I'm on my own because my shrink, who I saw recently, really thinks I should continue researching online because it's hard for me to come into their office and reach their demands...no car, no public transportation, and no license either. So I'm only seeing her it seems with my shared Medical Transportation which I share with each doctor I see, and each visit is 2 trips taken away. I only get 24 round trips in a year.

I will discover more in April when I come in for a Treatment Plan to see if they want me to have a therapist or really just the shrink. That's when I'm going to tell my STORY again there.You would think my story would be in their files. I've been going there on and off since 2004. When I moved I went to other therapists and other shrinks at other locations, but they didn't work out well...so that is why, I went back to my OLD place again where I am currently at. I'm familiarized with them more because I've been going there for so long.

It just seems the HELP isn't there. So, I'm the type of person who will investigate any topic when I'm curious to learn. So right now, my main focus is: ME, picking up the pieces and use what I can to grow. Peace & <3 to all! Remember, NEVER EVER GIVE UP!! :D

Loretta Ayers
USA

Little Girl

A little girl I see
Scared and alone
Cast aside because of disabilities
Left to hold her own
No friends to play with
The children laugh instead
They always seem to dismiss
Her accomplishments misread
They focus on things she can't change
Her eyes turn, she has a limp
They always have nasty words to exchange like freak, spazz, or gimp
They say the world would be a better place if she were to die
Oh yes, the world is cruel little girl
For she is only nine years old, contemplating suicide

Shawnna Hastings-Downey
Canada

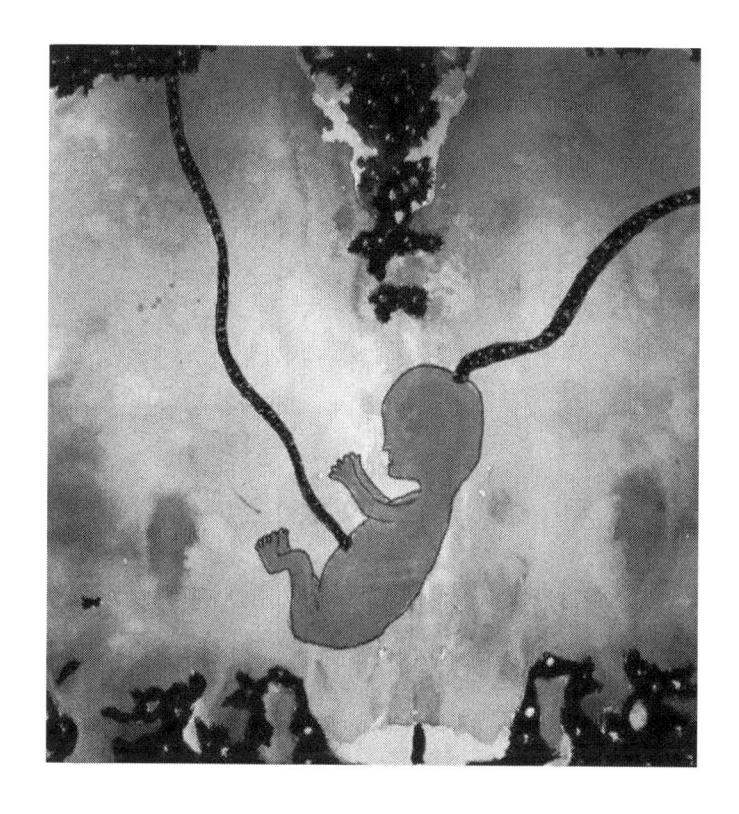

Dissociative Space Travel

Mal Hultgren
Sweeden

Hands wandering,
Mouths slobbering,
Fingers pointing,
Soul destroying

Inside burning
Stomach churning
Dry eyes crying
Slowly dying

Silent screams
Fists clenched
Heart pounding
Broken dreams

Hot breath
Deadly stare
Dirty smile
No one cares

Skin crawling
Now he's moaning
Hide my eyes
Hide my face
Take me away from this place.

One last thrust..
He's done
It's done
I'm done

Kirsty McCarthy
Wales

Every morning, I wake up and I absorb the lack of your love. I am nourished by your contempt, by your hopeless sighs, by the rolling of your eyes, by your enthusiasm for anything but me.

Your looks, your eyes, your voice are a judgment casting court. You don't know that, but I can feel it even before it happens.

I carefully listen to your words; I deconstruct them and keep them close to my heart, to my stomach, to my head. I absorb your contempt, and, all day long, I make nourishment out of it.

That's what nourishes me, what guides me through the night, what influences my choices. That's the way I choose to treat myself, to mistreat myself, to stop existing, to cover up my bursts and mortify my skin.

My actions used to be poised, controlled, premeditated, analyzed until they rolled on themselves, but they are now violent slaps against my face.

And I look for love where I shouldn't; I undress myself and I show my chains to those who find pleasure in hitting me again. I wish I had love - a great amount of love, unfathomable love, exaggerated love. I wish I had love, but my nudity is like fresh meat at the mercy of a hungry wolf. I show my blood to whoever is thirsty, to whoever is ready to eat up my suffering to satisfy his own absence. That's how they crush me, and I get crushed, and I crush myself.

And, once again, I live those mornings when I wake up and absorb the lack of your love. I swallow up more absence, more contempt, more humiliation. Today, this is who I am. An empty shell waiting to be filled but that doesn't know fulfillment, that is used to be crushed, again and again, that cannot resist the temptation of being reduced to dust.

Eleonora Nappi
Italy
Translated by Ombretta Di Dio

The (in)visible signs of sexual violence

"No visible signs of sexual violence."

I had the guts to use the word "rape" for the first time, referring to what G. did to me, during a conversation about sex. I was talking to a guy. He told me, "Ok, although it's not like he tied you or put a handkerchief in your moth. He didn't threaten you with a weapon." With those words, he was really testing the hard and patient work I had done on myself during all those months.

To be fair, G. really hadn't done any of that. He hadn't hit me, threatened me, nor had he used immobilizing objects. To be completely honest, he hadn't done anything besides ignoring my rejections, my prayers and my tears. And, besides denying myself with words, imploring him to stop while I was crying, I hadn't done anything either. I hadn't kicked, and I hadn't bitten. I hadn't screamed, and I hadn't tried to escape.

And this wasn't the only reason why that word – rape - lost its credibility. Yet it wasn't doubtful and uncertain anymore, it was almost self-aware while my mouth stronly pronounced it. G. hadn't been a stranger, nor what one would call a criminal. On the contrary, he was a person I used to love and with whom I had shared incredible moments. Sure, I probably cherished those moments much more than he did, but he claimed, and sometimes proved, to love me. At least, that's what I wanted to believe.
I can't exactly remember or define the moment I became so vulnerable, so easily manipulated and incapable of defending myself. What I perfectly remember, however, are the details of the day mutual consensus changed from granted, past element of our sexual relations to unimportant and unnecessary detail.

In order for us to elaborate a tragedy, however, someone other than us needs to sometimes see and deconstruct it. To accept and admit we have suffered an injustice, it is necessary for the injustice to be recognized as such by another human being. Someone who could act as a mirror to our feelings and confirm that our thoughts can be universally shared, and not merely interpreted with the filter of those emotions we have learned not to trust.

How could I claim to have been raped? Drunk women, women in short skirts, women who didn't show any sign of violence were often considered partly responsible for what happened to them. Their injustice would be undermined and not even considered as such by the majority of those men who were ready to decide what line shouldn't be crossed in consensual relationships. As if that was something you could talk about – an opinion – and not, instead, an obvious truth. How could I be considered a victim of rape when I knew my abuser, when I had loved him, desired him, when his sexual company had precedently given me ardent pleasure?
I never pressed charges against G. He still works hard, and he is largely respected and admired. His relationships are shallow and promiscuous. Recently, that part of me that stilll considers him as a companion with whom I once shared happy memories pushed me to look for him. I asked him whether he ever thinks about what happened between us. He laughed at me, and he told me I must be suffering from some sort of midlife crisis, since I constantly think about my past.

His life goes on. His persona remains solid, hard as a rock, deaf, closed to the contact with his emotional side and with the pain of others. He hasn't been affected in the least by those episodes which changed me dramatically. Maybe, one could truly say "no signs of violence were found" on him. A dark hole lies between us. We are strangers. We don't even belong to the same planet anymore.

I didn't do anything, and that's why I had not right to consider myself a victim. I was guilty of the injustice I had suffered. Since I was a child, I was taught that people hurt me because I was dumb, weak, and incapable of defending myself. The same was now true and confirmed by those around me. I hadn't done anything because I loved G, and I wished for him to love me too.

For once, I wanted him to hug me, to hold me tight without the underlying desire to penetrate me. Just for once. Then, we would have made love the way we did before: with passion, delicacy, strength, impetuosity.

Looking at each other in the eyes. I would have never been a static mean for pleasure, an empty shell, a toy in his rude and selfish hands. Instead, I would have been the passionate lover I had always been.

That's why I didn't do anything. He was the same person who made me feel protected and safe, and, since he constantly saw me cry and suffer, I couldn't stop thinking that he was going to eventually stop masturbating through my body.

"No visible signs of sexual violence."

I have read, heard, repeated these words that delicately curve my lips in a bitter smile.

I think of the theatricality of the body, of how those who suffer feel the necessity to show their pain. A necessity that often comes from a social need for blood, bruises, disease, evidence and immodesty. Injustices need to be visible and hurt the eyes. They need to upset our retinas, forcing us to move our eyes away, making it impossible for us to stare. However, not all rape victims show visible inner or external signs of violence. Sometimes, the violence is not visible or tangible.

"Violent" is an often misused adjective. It causes me to shake my head and smile with resignation. Just like "rude," "selfish," or "insensitive." Some words are never properly used in their right, real, and original meaning. Words, love, emotions, loneliness are what violence is, but – above all – hunger is violent.

Honestly, I sometimes think people do me a favor by slapping me.

"No visible signs of sexual violence."

I hug my ribs and I feel my throat burning. I know none of this is visible enough. The light, bitter smile on my face vanishes. I see hard work ahead of me. I need to show the signs. Someone needs to see my pain. I will be this way able to feel it, to engage in it, to stop hiding it and pushing it away and flushing it down the toilet. If someone sees me, I will start existing. I will be able to raise my eyes, to talk and tell my story without the incessant fear of being judged, teased, blamed.

Eleonora Nappi
Italy
Translated by Ombretta Di Dio

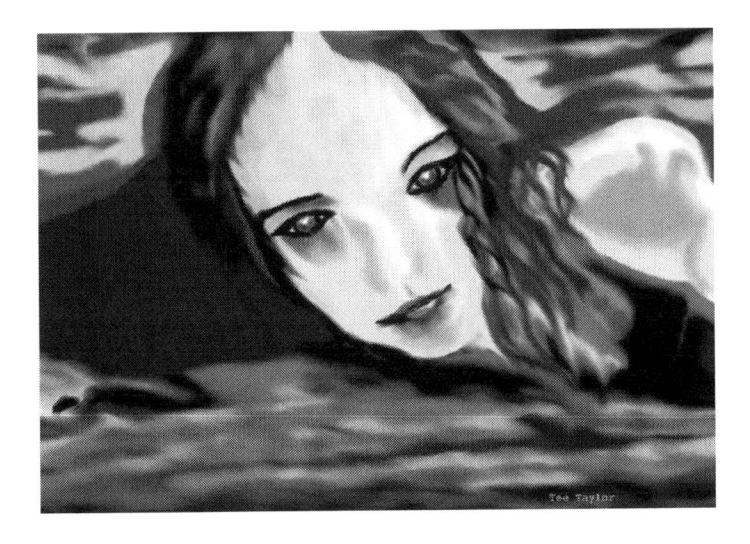

Against the Tide

Tee Taylor
UK

Scars Upon the Heart

If I told you how I feel, where would I start?
I'd tell you that there are scars upon my heart
If I dug deep down, what would I see?
Something discoloured, mutilated, and ugly
Scars left over from invisible wounds
The truth about bullying I will exhume
You may think that bullying is no big deal
But to some, it is terrifying and still seems real
Abuse in any form can be quite traumatic
In fact, it can create thoughts, feelings, and beliefs that are problematic
I have suffered through emotional abuse
And the things it caused me to believe would put some through a loop
Make them do a double take
Make them realize that the long term effects of bullying are not fake
I speak out about my scars to shed some light
On the damage that can be done, the damage that isn't in sight
Even though it's something you cannot see
It does not mean it's make believe
To be so young, contemplating death
Can be a very hard thing to accept
So I hid it away for many years
Hid the pain, hid the tears
And when they were finished, it was too late
You wonder how a little girl can have so much hate
For herself, for others, for the world around her
Why does negativity always surround her?
Because they took my feelings of joy, they threw them away
How can you defend yourself, when you have nothing left to say?
I admit, I'm lucky to have survived my tragic ordeal
But, that tragedy infused itself with my identity; that is how I truly feel

Shawnna Hastings-Downey
Canada

To: A Child Abuser, From: A Survivor

Dear Child Abuser,

First off, I want you to know that I survived. You may have broken me, but you did not shatter me completely. Secondly, please know that I realize that you too, suffer from a mental illness. I realize your actions are likely a response to the trauma you have suffered, likely as a child as well. I know somewhere inside of you there is a part of you that is so sick and twisted that perpetrating these acts of horror have somehow become your comfort and your sense of "normal". Perhaps there is even a part of you that wishes you had control over your actions, and maybe, just maybe you don't want to inflict the same pain that you suffered, but you lack the support you need to get well. That being said, I can forgive you to a point because you are sick, but I can never forget, and I hope if you ever read this you will realize the full extent of the damage you have caused me, and perhaps reach for help and not for a victim.

I am mentally sick also, however, you are a great deal of the reason I am sick. The difference between you and I, is I have not inflicted my illness onto others the way you have done to me, and so many others. Allow me to elaborate and let these words resonate in your mind.

You stole from me two things that can never be replaced...my innocence and my childhood. The ability to smile, laugh and play freely among my peers, snatched away and replaced with a shadow of overwhelming darkness. The sun didn't shine as bright, the birds songs, not so sweet and the first piece of me was lost and tucked away in a dark cave to be dealt with at another time. You took my ability to trust...both then and now. You made me question everyone that came into my life and cast a shadow of doubt on their intentions. You crushed my self esteem. You made me believe I was worth nothing. That I was so unloveable that you showing me your "love" was the closest I would ever get to love...and being under 8 years old, I believed you. You made me believe I would never amount to anything, and that it was my fault it was happening because "that's what little girls like you deserve for being bad". You instilled a sense of guilt and shame that I struggle with to this day. Infact, there is not an aspect of my life, from my relationships to my ability to work, that you have not affected. I will never have normal relationships, or the full ability to trust, the ability to love and be loved, all destroyed by your touch.

Now let me tell you something. As much as you destroyed me, you made me stronger. You made me empathetic to others, you made me strong enough to stop the destructive cycle with me. You made me realize that although you touched my body, over and over, you did not touch my soul. I was physically there but I mentally escaped to a safe place where people like you simply don't exist. My body has long healed from your scars, my mind not so much...but it will one day, because I will not allow you any more control over my life. I cannot take back what you ripped away from me, but I can stand up and tell you, I survived you and your illness, and I will survive and thrive from the illness you have inflicted on me. You will not have the last word, you will not control one more minute of my life. You have given me the power to have a voice, to stand up and tell people what you did, and do my best to fight for the children who have yet to find their strength to speak. My words may not resonate with you, but they will for the rest of us...the survivors that can not be broken by your illness.

I beg you to seek help in any way you possibly can. I know you are hurting like me, but you do have a choice NOT to hurt others....I have made that choice, and I hope one day you will too.

Many things in life can be fixed or replaced, the loss of childhood innocence is not one of them.

Jody Betty
Canada

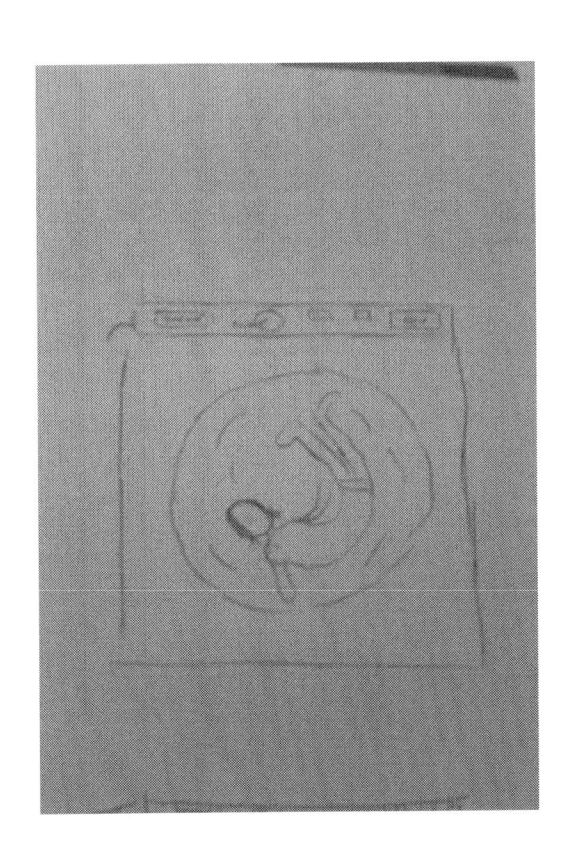

The Never ending Cycle

Amy Jennings
UK

"My name is Liliana."

When I was a little girl, I was gutted and emptied by the people I loved the most. The only way I could survive was to cause a death of self. I'm nothing but a mangled, tender and open wound of a girl. I have been turned inside out and I feel everything and everyone. A vessel for things to come in and out of but nothing stays. I can't see myself reflected anywhere. So, I'll be you & you & you, anything but me. I have no self to return to and I have no where to be. It's hard for me to stay in one place for long, I'm constantly shifting.

I'm diagnosed with Borderline Personality Disorder, Bipolar II, Post Traumatic Stress Disorder and Social Anxiety. My body has been raped, pinched, punched, slapped and spat on. I have scars all are over my body, some are visible and others are not. I have been told I'm too sensitive, dramatic, fragile and that I need to "let it go". My real name has become tainted. _____, you are a bitch, liar, slut and a whore. I'm so use to violence, darkness and pain, that anything light seems unreal. Love is both my haven and cause for my suffering and self-sabotage. I desire to be loved and to feel safe. I hold onto love so tightly and anxiously, that I end up crushing it into dust. My heart is a graveyard for everyone I ever loved. They're ghosts and constantly haunting me, reminding me that I'm absolutely terrible.

I see my death everywhere. Stepping into traffic, falling off the balcony, stabbing myself and electrocuting myself in the bathtub. I don't want to leave my bed because I'm so afraid I will do it. Deep down I don't want to die but I'm afraid it would happen. I remember the worst depression I experienced was when I was in a abusive relationship. I started taking everything less seriously. I felt insignificant. I even tattooed the word on my left index finger. Just to remind myself, it doesn't matter and I don't either. I stopped doing simple things like bathing, doing my laundry and eating. I felt so heavy and I'd rot in bed, day after day. I wouldn't even sleep.

I didn't have the energy to go to the bathroom. I had cups I'd keep by my bed to urinate in. I attempted suicide by swallowing a handful of pills. I was tired of existing in other people's stories but not my own. I was tired of the silence within myself. I was tired and sick of myself.

I carry so much shame and guilt inside myself. I have difficulty saying no and setting boundaries. This often leads me to disastrous and traumatizing events. I don't feel I have the right to myself and most times, I think I deserve whatever I get. So, I freeze and let it happen. I've had so many people have sex at me but not with me. I've always thought if I gave too much, eventually someone will see me. I have an overwhelming desire to be understood. It doesn't matter though, it won't matter who I am or how much I give of myself if it's to the wrong people.

When I was a little girl, this isn't the life I dreamed of for myself. I'm still a little girl in a lot of ways and I've been stumbling throughout life in that perspective. I had plans for this body of mine and now it works against me. I imagine myself as one of those Matryoshka dolls, each layer revealing another until nothingness. My pain isn't visible and the depths to which I feel are uncomprehending.

The only thing that gives me any sense of hope these days is,

Beautiful things can come from the wounds we bare and where there is emptiness, it is merely a blank space for creation. "

Liliana Beth Reckless
Canada

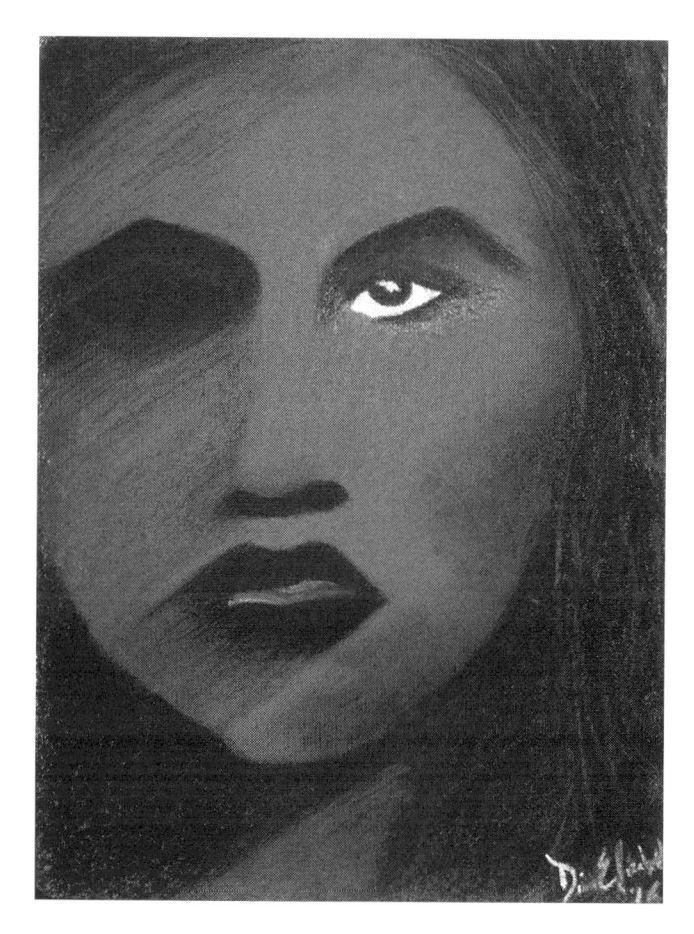

Disintegration of Self

Dion Elizabeth
USA

My story...

I was born in 1979 daughter of a miner, an only child but 5 step brothers and sisters I grew up with. It was Thatcher Year's. My dad was made redundant. His pay was quite high. He bought our house then 2 others and let them out. We were pretty well off. I had all the latest designer clothes on. We pretty much travelled the world over the next couple of years. So my mum and dad had the money to sit in the pub all day... I was about 11 then I'd grew up pretty normal.

Only me and my brother still lived at home. Then my older brother Anthony got cancer. He had treatment and went into remission and moved into a bedsit opposite of our house.

Eleven was a difficult age for me. I was a fat kid, didn't have any confidence, so I used to go and sit with Anthony. He had had a troubled life. We used to talk about how different we were from the rest of the family. I used to go to church with him. He confided in me he'd been raped. I was the only living person that knew, made us closer.

Then my brothers Anthony, his cancer had come back. He was only 23.... He was living in our front room on a special bed, and as close as we were, I just felt weird watching him fade away. He'd just lie with his bible as though that would cure him.

I became angry. I started hanging around with the wrong people. At 12 my boyfriend was a 17yr old drug dealer that I thought was amazing. All my mates were getting drunk and slagging about how I had intimacy issues, always have. I only feel comfortable with body contact with certain people. I thought that was just me, so I did what the boys did. I was taking acid, mushrooms, amphetamines, weed, fuck it. Mum and dad are probably drunk or up all night with Anthony. I just lived in the same house, no one had any idea.

The cancer finished him off quickly. Anthony went into the hospice. I had tonsillitis so wasn't allowed in. I didn't see him for his last 10 days. I never got to say goodbye. We were supposed to be going to Africa together and doing Christian missionaries work. We were just gonna go off on our own where we felt comfortable. I know it sounds weird because of the age gap, but out of all 5 he was the only one who understood me. I went to see his body. He was still warm. I was so close to my goodbye, but all the cancer had started turning purple. I didn't want to walk out the room.

The funeral came, it was just a blur. My brother who still lived at home collapsed in a mess. The church was rammed. Everyone was comforting everyone. I just stood against the wall and watched. I was 12.

I'd been grabbed by a man with a knife 2 weeks before the funeral. But that I kept locked away. I escaped. He punched me in the crotch. The police caught him but his friend gave him an alibi. He was even seen lurking where he jumped out at me 10 minutes before he actually did.

But I can't think about it.

Anthony tried to comfort me one of the last times I seen him. He understood. He'd been there. I pushed him away... I got on with life.

Mum and dad's days in the pub were getting more and more regular. It was at the stage I'd have to go to the pub to get a con from the bar, or given money to make myself scarce. That was my tea, so I'd go out, latest trainer's loads of money I was a spoilt brat to everyone.

Then, when I had to be in at 9, I'd go back to the Pub and wait for them to go home unless Michael was in, which wasn't often. He was a chef. So I'd sit there listening to conversation's I really shouldn't have been hearing getting the odd beer brought me.

189

Then when we did finally go home I went to bed my mum and dad would have sex so loud I could hear what they were saying, or fight. I have a few childhood memories of coming down in the middle of the night and see my dad throttling my mum or giving her a backhander. I just used to go back to bed into my world again.

But now I was old enough to understand my mum's screaming. I had to go down. This carried on in a blur till I was 15. I honestly cannot remember much of them years. I was out clubbing, selling drugs with a boyfriend too old for me. I would never sleep. And I finally clicked why my mum and dad never did too. I mean drinking all day shagging or arguing all night. They were taking drugs too... I did get a few hours sleep before school sometimes. But no one bothered. Never got questioned about homework. No one gave a fuck, why should I?

School never even questioned me. No one knew. I was in the latest clothes. I had money. How could I be neglected? I'd not lived in a family home for many years, it was 2 people getting fucked up on drugs with a daughter who did the same to forget what she had to go home to. If I did go home. I stayed here, there, and everywhere. Grown men's houses. Never questioned...Then things became really fucked up!

My best friend who was a couple of years younger than me started seeing a 26yr old boy racer. Fuck that. I wasn't getting in that nonsense car. So I started hanging around with my mate's brother. He was well known for being hard at it with the drugs. We got together 3 days before my 16th birthday.

I had money thrown at me. We used to buy drugs and just stay at home. My mum and dad were never in till the early hours. And my dad started buying big quantities of amphetamine and used to give me and him some. The night before my final English exam my dad gave my fella some fet for me. I went to the exam with no sleep and completely fucked up.

Why didn't anyone notice who I was or what I was doing? Because nobody cared. I wasn't worthy of love. I learned that when I was about just 13.

I wasn't like my mum and sister. When we went out I'd have jeans and boots on and they'd be in mini skirts and see through tops. I was the fat boring one with big boobs. Or the bitch, as my mum often referred to me after she'd had a drink.

We'd come home from the pub quite early. I'd been sat outside crying in a doorway. I just wanted to go home with no arguments, or better still I wish my mum and dad weren't sat in that pub out their faces. I needed Anthony. When they seen I had been crying they come home through embarrassment of me crying and people seeing me.

My mum wanted to get in the pub early so she had forgot to go shopping. I called her a cow. First time I ever cussed my parents. I watched through my brother's bedroom window as my dad consoled my mum. She was a brilliant mum and I was being a cow…it was me. Was my fault. I felt heartbroken though to see my mum cry so I vowed from that day any hurt she caused me I would just keep in. I don't want to make her cry again.

We moved into a pub. I was 16. I had old men leering at me, telling me they're gonna sniff my pants. Got offered 200 cigs for a blow job by a man who could've been my granddad. My mum thought it was all funny. She used to encourage me to do drinking races with the locals. I'd win she'd get free beer.

Then mum and dad lost everything. They'd drunk and snorted it all. They were bankrupt on benefits. I was a 17 year old wreck, half the size I used to be. We lived in a mould ridden flat that aggravated my asthma. I couldn't face being trapped just with them two. I had no choice. I was penniless, a mess.

Mum and dad liked my boyfriend, a 28 year old married man. We just partied. I got pregnant but miscarried after I caught my fella in bed with my friend. I moved back in with mum and dad. I got a day and night job so I was never there. Then I got back with him, but stayed with my parents.

One night I went to see him. He was in bed with her again. I wasn't pregnant this time. All the hurt from losing the baby came out. I picked up a plank of wood, knocked him out, and broke all but 1 of her ribs. I got arrested. Sentenced to 2 months in jail, which wasn't as bad as the 18 months that carries for my crime.

I was lead away to jail at 18yrs old. It was scary as hell. My 1st night on suicide watch in a ward with a view of some fat woman's arse who was on her period. Blood everywhere. The opposite way, a schizophrenic girl was arguing with someone in the bathroom who wasn't there. I cried till daylight.

I met a girl who was from my town. She knew my fella. She watched over me. I learned how to tell people to fuck off, which did me good! Got released then went back to my jobs and mum and dad's. They were really fucked up.

My mates used to come round and we'd take drugs. Mum and dad would take them with us. Then my dad started having psychosomatic delusions. We'd all be sitting there, then my dad would jump up shouting. He said he'd been watching us all wink all night arranging for my mum to have sex with my 19yr old friend. It was madness. He said we all knew and kicked everyone out at like 5am. Then I just tried to hide in my bedroom, but he kept coming in saying look just admit it I won't be mad, over and over he wouldn't leave me alone. I think I finally fell asleep to wake up to him still having mum sat on sofa going on about it. It scared the shit outta me.

Then over the next few months it got hard. He said we were trying to kill him. Or we were drugging him up so men could come and have sex with mum. We'd spend days locked in this argument. He was convinced. He had us both in a room shouting we were slags, and we weren't allowed out for tampering with evidence he was looking for. Once he had us outside explaining some mud on a window sill. That one went on for days.

One morning he came in and woke me up shouting at me to get out that fuckin bed now. I was like wtf. I only had underwear on. I was crying. I didn't want to because I was in my pants, but he come to whip covers off me. So I slid them off. He thought I had a man hidden in my bed for my mum to have sex with. That's when I knew I had to get away. They were fuckin my head in.

So who did I go back to...

We got married when I was 18. On the day of our wedding we were on MDMA. He went off and brought some girls to the reception. Then his best man got photos out of my husband licking the stripper's pussy he'd had the night before.

My mum and dad were on a come down. They'd not slept; been awake arguing all night. They just sat in a corner arguing on more drugs.

We got our flat. I worked on and off like him. He often spiked me. Drugs were getting bad for him. He was hanging round with an old friend who was a smackhead. One Wednesday, I walked in from work to find they'd smoked all my weed, which I smoked to calm me or I didn't eat or sleep. Two smackheads were sat monged out with needles still hanging out of em.

That's it. It clicked I had to get away or that would've been me, so I got a bag of clothing and my 2 cats at walked out at 11pm. Never went back! But now I was 21 homeless 2 cats and had my dad's the only place to go...

I settled into my dad's, started a degree to be a teacher, and worked part time. My mum and dad had just split up before I moved back in so things were pretty shitty. It came to his birthday so I took him out for a drink. I met this bloke playing pool, not much to look at if I'm honest, but he was the opposite of my husband. Seemed outgoing, charming. So I agreed a date.

1st July. He took me out, charmed me, said all the things I wanted to hear. We got serious. He left his Mrs and kids to be with me, but I didn't even know of them till I was in too deep. So I made him pick. He did me.

We spent all our time together, and after a while he started going to pool on his own so I arranged a night out with a few mates. We didn't go anywhere, stayed in and took ecstasy instead. Me and 3 mates, 2 were male but only friends. We were having a brilliant night. I thought he was pooling, then I got a knock at the door. It was him. I let him in the porch but wouldn't let him in the house. My mates were battered and he was kicking off big time.

That was the first time he scared me a bit. After an hour arguing. He went. But things had changed drastically. He would ring me through the day asking who I was with, where, and where was I going next. Every time we went out to bars I couldn't speak to any bloke he didn't know. When we got home he would argue about me flirting with someone or being in toilet too long.

Then my brother the chef booked his wedding in the Dominican Republic. Me and dad booked our tickets to go. By now mum had remarried and dad had met someone. So that shit with them wasn't so bad. I told Martin about the wedding and I was going. He said if I went he would set fire to my mum's bungalow while she was in bed. We argued. I said don't be ridiculous. He said leave the country and try me! So that was me not going to my brothers wedding.

I didn't realize it at the time, but I'd started trying to do everything to appease him. I didn't wear make up in the day. I stopped going out with friends, all to save arguments. Then one night we went out. We'd had a tiff before so there was an odd atmosphere between us. Anyway I got drunk. So did he. We got home, and again I was flirting with someone, or I did this or that. Anything. I think he used to watch me all night to find excuses sometimes, but things got heated he grabbed me and shook me. I lashed out knocking his arms off me, then we grappled. I ended up laid on the floor, him stood over my head with a two foot ceramic vase ready to drop on my face.

I just got up in time, but I had 3 massive like holes in my arms. Not big, just deep. He freaked out tried to help me up. I told him to fuck off. That enraged him again. He was chasing me round our flat, grabbing and pulling at me. I grabbed the phone, rung 999, he ripped the cord out the wall. I just had to keep running away.

Blood was just splashing everywhere. I was holding my cuts, but they were too far apart for me to cover them all. He finally caught me at the top of our stairs to our 2nd storey flat, at the end of our hall in front of the window. He's got both his hands round my neck telling me he was going to fuckin kill me, he was just shouting. I couldn't hear. I was frozen with fear. Then out the corner of my eye I see out the window police cars pulling up. I had to just stay calm so he wouldn't see my reaction to the police coming, let go, and fill them with bullshit.

Six officers ran up my stairs. They grabbed him off me and literally dragged him so he fell down the stairs. A lady officer escorted me in the front room asked what my injuries were. I told her my black eye, bruised neck, and cuts on my arm. She asked where did all the blood come from. It was on every wall in every room as I was running away. I just explained. She asked a little about what happened then got me in an ambulance.

Martin came to the hospital to get me before I could be seen. The cuts were just seeping for 2 days. He wouldn't let me go back to hospital. Finally he agreed to take me to the nurse. She injected the anaesthetic straight into the holes to numb it. The pain was unreal. I was crying. He made me say I fell over on a glass.

He stood over me and the nurse all the way through. No emotion just staring, making the odd polite gesture. I was sewn up, 13 stitches in 3 holes about 2-3 cm across. They had to pull the skin back together they'd been open so long.

Life carried on.

I couldn't believe what an epic fail I'd had at sorting my life out, was supposed to be a teacher. Quite habitual use of class A's, working. Then I met him. We carried on. Him controlling where and when I go anywhere apart from work, he didn't like that. But he was better about work than college. Had to quit that, too many men.

I'd started thinking this was all I was worth. Damaged goods from all the shit I still carried in my head between mum and dad. And most of all still no Anthony. Fuck it. I'll settle for what I am now.

I used to listen to Pink's song 'Just Like a Pill' a lot! It was my life there and then. Then one day at work I fell downstairs. Hurt my tendons. First aider took me to a&e, but for some reason I just knew I couldn't have an x-ray till I'd done a pregnancy test. Till that moment it hadn't even occurred to me I was pregnant. So I went home.

My mum's new husband brought me some tests. Positive. When I told Martin I thought he was going to pass out. Well I'd had polycystic ovaries, endometriosis and 3 miscarriage behind me. I was put through the hormonal change after I'd just got married to try restart everything and not miscarry again. I'd not been pregnant since. So I assumed I was well messed up and never gonna be a mum.

Which is all I'd wanted after Anthony. The same unconditional love. My family had very certain conditions to show any love or protection and hadn't done for many years. So a baby. Mine to love and cherish, and most of all love me because no one else did. But I'd also accepted I wasn't a proper woman. So the positive line on there changed everything.

I carried on at work light duties. I felt so good. I'd had no pain or blood like before. Went for my 12wk 1st scan, my sister was with me. Martin had to work? She put the thing on my belly. There was my pregnancy sac measuring right but no baby. It's called a blighted ovum, Latin for fated egg. The body's way of getting rid of an abnormal pregnancy. They wanted me to stay in that night to operate and remove the pregnancy sac. But I went home. I laid on my dad's sofa and sobbed all night.

Next morning had my op. Woke up in agony, and a terrible lonely feeling. My bump had gone. Martin come running in ward and started crying all over me. I didn't feel anything for him. He'd not lost it. I just disconnected from everything for quite a while. Then a few months later I got the feeling again. I'm pregnant. So I did a test. Positive. I was happy, scared, excited, and then I'd think of my baby's dad.

But I wanted this baby more than anything. Things progressed good. My 1st scan again. Mum was with me. There she was, my baby, kicking away. From then on I concentrated on the baby. Martin still use to come in drunk and hit me, but it would be on the legs where no one seen.

He used to make me sleep on the sofa 8 months pregnant. I was massive. It was long nights on there. Not quite sure why he did now, but I'd spend 3 or 4 nights a week on there easy. One Sunday I felt a trickle. My waters, thank God. Two weeks late.

I ended up being at home in slow labour for 2 days before they took me in to speed things up. That was a Monday morning at 7am. I was given every drug going, but she didn't wanna come out.

Martin kept dropping in, but didn't stay. I later learned he went to the pub to meet his knock off. Finally, I delivered her Wednesday morning at 1:15 am. A huge 60cm 9lb 4half oz. She was gorgeous.

We went home. I had to learn to be a mummy, which I loved. Martin was still drinking and hitting me, but I was taking it so she had her dad. I had a black eye every other week. I didn't always ring the police. Sometimes it was easier to take it so I could get some sleep.

He punched me in the face once whilst breastfeeding, I did ring the police. My cousin was a police officer at the time and just by chance he was the one to come. I gave a statement. Martin was ringing me from different public phone boxes asking if the police were there still and could he come home. The police were instantly tracking the calls and sending officers he was running all over town. It was like a wild goose chase, but they got him. He was locked up but released on bail the next day.

He came back all apologetic and promised it will never happen again. I believed him and dropped the charges. Things carried on, he kept hitting me. He once leaned over our baby who was in bed with me to spit at me and hit me. I just rolled over her and lay in front of her to protect her and took my slap, then he let me sleep again.

Police got called again one night. I can't even remember why. But he had smashed the flat up. His bail conditions were to stay away from me. Our flat was just in his name so legally I had to move out. I found a house. He weedled his way back in. Decorating, playing nice guy, he'd not hit me for a few weeks....

He then lost the flat we'd shared...

He'd pretty much moved in, but it was nearly Christmas so I thought for Jessica's first he was being ok. It could work. It did for a while, then abuse started crawling back in. Name calling, telling me I was useless, no one would ever have me.

Then one Saturday at the beginning of May we arranged for Jess to stay with my mum. And me and him were going out alone. God forbid I ever go out without him. But he decided he wanted to go to the pub that afternoon. He came back at 7pm bladdered. Demanding me to suck his dick. He had raped me once before. I didn't tell anyone. I was too ashamed. But my friend came round a couple of days after, and she was like wtf happened to you. I told her. She immediately started taking photos of the black eyes, bruised cheek, and a nasty horrible love bite all round my neck. I buried that shit with the man who attacked me. That's in a bit of my brain I leave untouched.

Anyway, him demanding a blow job triggered that, and I thought not again, so I went in the next room and put the sofa up to the door while he was lay on my baby's sofa shouting profanities.

When he realized I wasn't playing ball, I had no Jess I could finally be braver, he started demanding my money to go back to the pub. He started getting aggressive saying to give him the fuckin money. So he said I'll just get it out your purse, which was in the barricaded front room with me.

He come to walk in and realized what I'd done so he couldn't get at me. He went berserk. He rammed the door and the sofa halfway across the room and grabbed me somehow. I was on the floor with him sat over me shouting something at me then banging my head on the floor. I think I passed out because the next thing I knew he was stood up getting my purse. I just legged it upstairs. He threw a massive glass ashtray at me, which caught my heels. As I was 2 steps away from the top I just run into the bedroom.

I was trapped.

He jumped at me then sat on top of me trapping one arm, and with both fists just kept punching me in the face. I just tried to fend him off with my one hand scratching him and turning my face from side to side to minimize damage. He just stopped suddenly and run out the house. I looked in the mirror I realized why. My entire face was bruised, my eyes were swollen, my ears were 3 times the size and purple. Luckily my daughter was at my mum's so I cowered up on the sofa waiting for him to come back.

The next day I got a knock at the door. It was the police come to arrest me for assault on him, the scratches I did on his arm. They took one look at my face, radioed to station, then come and took a statement. I had to have forensics come take photos of me. He was charged with assault and battery, and he denied it. I had to endure crown court and the abuse of all his family even though it was him that actually rung the police.

I concentrated on Jess. One night we were having our nightly bath together, playing. I had the radio on and a song came on that hit me like a ton of bricks. It was Evanescence, "Bring Me To Life." As I listened, tongue words, it was like my subconscious telling me to listen. I did. I wasn't going to be a wreck that never went out.

I got a part time job and enrolled in accountancy college. I got on with my life. I was rebuilding for me and Jessica. He was sentenced to 15 months in prison. We carried on. That was 10 years ago. I buried it, moved on with my life, met my husband and got pregnant. We had a little boy.

My life should have been perfect. I got postnatal depression really bad. I was suicidal. I was hearing voices. I kept asking for help. No one did. They just gave me pills. Then I seen a cpn who changed my life. She took me to a specialist psychiatrist who diagnosed borderline personality disorder.

I had an answer why I'd always been different. I had psychotherapy. I got a lot out, but it was hard. I had lots of different tablets, a cpn. I muddled through life.

My husband's son start staying that it was hard merging a family.

Jess was growing up believing Andrew was her dad. She's always been a bugger. Then my mum died. She got took to hospital one day and we got told she had 48 hours to live. Lewis was only 5 months old. My head totally fucked up all the stuff I'd come to terms with. I never got chance to say, "Mum why did you encourage me to be promiscuous and drink when I was a child." Why did she once give a man outside a bar a blow job for £5 in front of me? But it all died with her.

My husband was amazing. He took so much grief. I would run out the house, flip out, disassociate, but he stayed. I was finally thinking maybe he loved me. I tried my best to deal with the grief. Jess really struggled. We took her to an amazing charity who helped bereaved children, it helped. We all muddled on. Lewis was my ray of sunshine.

Then Jess's psychologist said we should tell her about her real dad. Between ages of 8 + 10 we did. She accepted it. Life continued. I battle my head on a daily basis still. I disassociate. I have panic attacks. I won't go out the house for months. My own world I've always retreated to...

I left Jess to ask what she need, but her behaviour was becoming harder to deal with. Her dad got in touch with her on Facebook. I didn't know. She told me he invited her round to his new daughter's birthday party. I understood she would be curious and I tried to separate my feelings for hers. I was still grieving. I wasn't thinking straight. I've battled so hard to keep going. I've had 2 suicide attempts.

Over the years since mum's died dad still asks me about certain nights. Telling me my mum fucked him behind his back, or she'd done this, or I still knew about that. It was worse when I worked with him on the way home. He would bring mum up. She was dead, why? I had to tell him if it didn't stop I would have to disconnect myself to protect my mental health. He calmed down.

Mum's been dead 9 years this year. He still said something a couple of months ago about a man in a nearby village that I knew mum was seeing. I just have to live with it now. He's old, away with the fairies for all his medication, so now I'm the parent. I have to tell him it's inappropriate to talk about sex in front of my kids.

Once he come coked up. Told him he'd never see his grandkids again. I'm not having anyone on drugs around my kids. At least my parents taught me, 'what not to do'.

Then a couple big years ago we had a surprise. We called her Amelia. She was born poorly on the 22nd December 2013. I lived in intensive care with her over Christmas while my husband was here trying to keep Christmas normal.

It was now we realised how bad Jessica had become. I came home to see them and the hospital rung for me to get there fast. Jess point blank refused to move anywhere. Since then she's smoked at 11, boys at 13, drugs, beer. We've had it all.

She's been under camhs, and as for two years now we know my daughter has traits of ADHS, ADD, and ODD. She runs away from home and went to stay with her dad once. Her social workers, the police, no one would do anything. That was this year.

From New Year's Eve, for about 3 weeks since, Jess has returned home. She shouts and screams at me that I lied about him hitting me so bad. I played the victim. He's told her his events of the past and makes him look like super dad. He told her I made him sign his parental responsibility away. The court gave that verdict because of his violence, and he didn't show up to hear that verdict.

I think so, it wasn't listed as his violence, but she believes everything he says, and when she has a meltdown she's always throwing it in my face. From then on I just shut down and replay every time he hit me. I'm cowering again.

Then last week my daughter really went for me. My husband had her in a bear hug for 10 minutes before she stopped trying to attack me. She said she wants to batter me because of the lies I've said about her dad. And today my daughter's social workers been after visiting him, and wants me and him to sit in a room and discuss Jess staying over.

Martin, him has said he won't do it unless I'm present. That's really set me off. I feel like I've got to prove to everyone what he did. My daughter has a cpn therapists and psychiatrist as well, no one will help me with it. Like I should take her attacks, but last time when she was coming at me for a minute I wanted to thrash her.

She's 14, same height and build as me, screaming at me I'm a lying fruitloop, my fear turned to anger. And that scares me. The police won't really do anything as said they will but that was 8 week ago.

I'm at my wits end. I wish I knew someone who has any advice or similar experiences, or knows how I can get his police record or my statements, anything. So he can't keep lying and trying to control me through Jess, and saying he won't do any meeting unless I'm there. I don't have to be. He's trying to control me still.

Everyone is telling me my daughter needs to be removed from the house for the safety of Lewis and Amelia. It's hard. I fought for her for so long, but I really am a broken woman. I'm 36 on mood stabilizer's, antidepressants, and diazepam for anxiety. That's been since my daughter started getting worse.

I can't cope...

On August 10th last year I nearly took my life again. Purely because I feel so alone. Although I have my husband, kids and my dad, sort of. Bless him. That's what living with borderline is like, you never know what's coming. Are you going to be depressed, or manic, or anxious, or scared because of all the thoughts in your head.

My son's teacher raised concerns he's autistic. So now I'm gonna be taking him for assessment and tests, and I think he's seen too much of Jess attacking me. Maybe he would be better without Jess here. Last week I went to my doctor and my 2 year old picked up we were talking about Jess and said, "Jess hit mummy and shout and banged door." Doctor looked at me as if to say that's heartbreaking. I'm torn. But I still continue to keep getting up going. That's what matters.

It's like borderline controls part of my mind. It makes me think things. I have to use the techniques I've learned over the years to conquer it. Sometimes I win; sometimes I lose...but I'm just about always alone. But I won't give up my fight... I can't...

Jolene Potter
UK

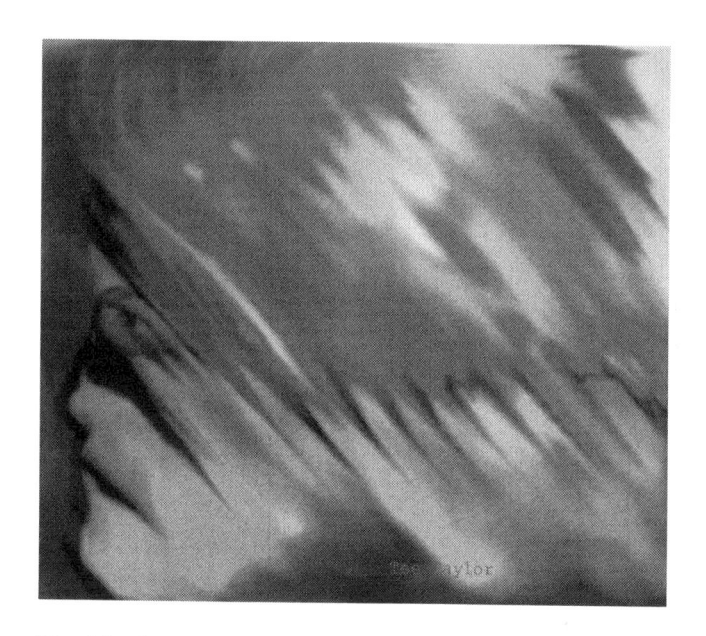

Untitled

Tee Taylor
UK

V.

Moments of Change

Moments of change can be minor or major depending where you are on your journey. Sometimes a moment of change is a glimmer of light in the darkness of your mind. Other times it hitting rock bottom and committing to wellness and recovery. Either way, moments of change are ones that take us from hopeless to hopeful.

Livia Richard
USA

Some things change you for good no matter how much you fight or how many positive changes you make you just can't seem to shake it.
It's like a dark shadow that only sees small moments of light bright enough to hide its evil existence, but it's still there just waiting for the light to dim enough so it can resurface and remind me of EVERYTHING!

Stacey Heaney
BPD Survivor
Australia

Letter to Building 18

I was there, letting him tell me it all, letting him describe and explain.

I was listening to the long list of her qualities, her false faults, all the nice things she did, how adorable it was when he hurt her, and what a shame it was that she wasn't expressing her full potential. Suddenly, the heartache was there again. Time, numbers, even the control of my own body was forgotten. A rush of sadness would come over me dragging me down. I could remember everything.

Ever since I was back, I stopped feeling. I once again started to weigh, measure, count, calculate and worry that everything would go according to my plans. My whole existence went by along intrusive numbers and nervous calculations, and I had no contact whatsoever with what Mr C. Defined as my life. He would tell me that, in talking about myself, I sounded like I was referring to somebody else.
I was perfectly aware of what I was afraid to feel and to remember, and, out of the blue, it was now falling all over me, tactless and unannounced, as if I had opened a packed closet letting its content fall over a motionless me.

What I wished – and I felt that right away – was for somebody to speak about me the way he spoke about her.

I wished someone would sit on a bench with a friend or a stranger and would proceed to enlist all of my qualities (or what he considered as endless qualities) and my funny faults as if those faults were nothing but an extension of my qualities. I wished someone would blush, with eyes and mouth opened in a silly smile, at the idea of my presence on this Earth. I wished for somebody's heart to be full and for somebody's hands to be shaky and I wished for that somebody to be happy. Basically, I wished somebody loved me.

Yet I always ran away when that possibility became slightly tangible. The thought of someone touching me so deeply and exposing me in such a way while cherishing me made me completely anxious. I didn't want to be that real.

And now that I was coming back to life by getting inevitably in touch with the most atrocious and painful things, what I wanted seemed out of reach and impossible. I couldn't foresee any second chance to escape a loneliness so violent and intolerable that it was now forcing me back to my calculations.

However, I took a heavy, radical and scary decision that day. I took a piece of paper and a pen and I wrote a letter that I thought would change my life.

"Dear Lucia,

I am writing this letter to let you know that I am choosing to leave this place.

Please, don't cry, don't wet the paper with your tears, don't mess it up with your bony hands, don't scream, don't yell, don't kick the ground, don't cut yourself, don't skip any meal, don't force yourself to throw up.

I am abandoning you Lucia, that much is true, but you need to learn to accept that.

This white place – with light pink walls – is designed to be a bubble, a happy oasis where nothing can affect us.

There is something you need to know, this bubble is a lie.

Even here, you see, there are people who are abandoning you.

The worst part is that you will have to learn how to live with it, because it will happen again, it will happen all the time, even here.

And while I will always be ready to read your letters, to answer to your calls and attend to your needs, you will understand that this will not always be possible and you will sometimes find a silent and hard wall in front of you.

You are allowed to cry, but not to come back to this place.

Protecting yourself from everything will not allow you to avoid all type of contact because, ultimately, human beings cannot avoid distress. It doesn't matter if you, my dear Lucia, feel like you are made to experience more pain than others while being capable of sustaining less. There are no facilitations for those who feel more.

Stay where you are because no place is really better than your own life, and the death you are so carefully faking will not give you what you are hoping to get.

Nothing will happen if you dare to eat that olive that you purposely left in your plate, Lucia. That won't destroy you.

That's simply life, and life is not something from which you should protect yourself.

You need to learn to feel your flesh grow: full, alive, loud and messy. That's how life is supposed to be. It's not as white, sparkly and sanitized as this room.

I know you can't really see what I am saying. My words are like blurry lines for those eyes filled with tears, for those ears so deaf to any invitation to change, for those legs always ready to jump up and down the hospital.

Still I know that you are not this frail, angry being who is ready to attack and who is now yelling at me while I leave the horizon.

I remember when you used to dream of doing things and you used to let people touch you. You wouldn't jump. You would simply stay where you were. You need to stay where you are. If you stay still, the storm will not wet you as much, and it will eventually stop. But you cannot avoid the storm.

I am sorry, but you have no choice."

But - I need to say that - I haven't given the letter to the sender yet.

I always see her, in the hallway number 18. Last time I saw her, somebody told her she had her dad's mannerisms, and when that happened, she came back to life. She smiled discreetly and she curiously and conceitedly asked where that resemblance came from.

She smiled, but she wasn't even aware of that.

I still hope I will be able to give her my letter, to sit on the other side, the side that belongs to the righteous saviors.

Apparently though, I am not believable enough.

Eleonora Nappi
Italy
Translated by Ombretta Di Dio

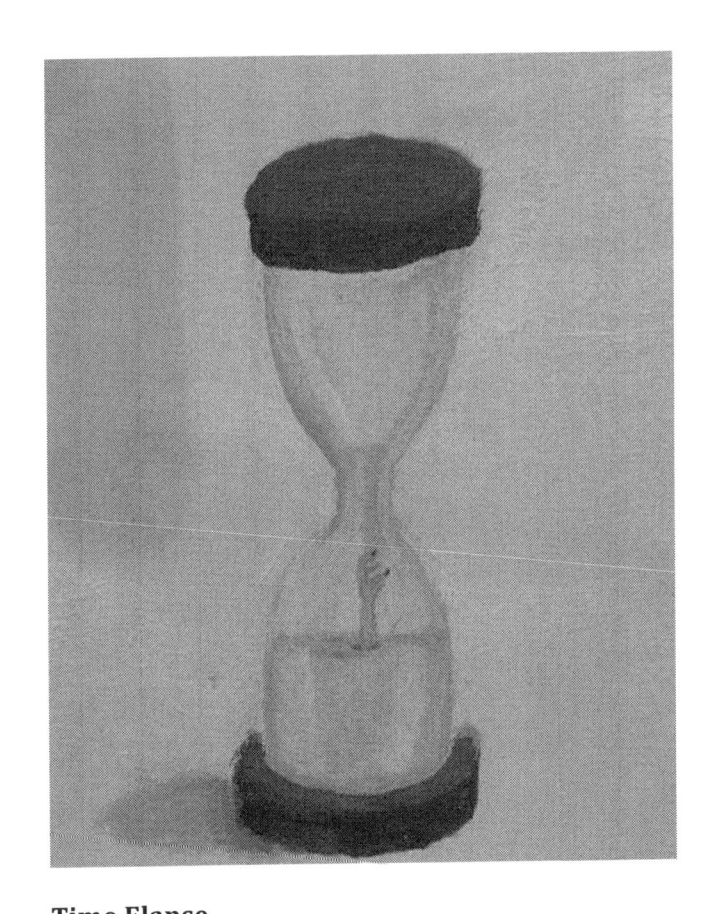

Time Elapse

Mal Hultgren
Sweeden

Finding My Feet Again

The cracks in the day began in the early hours of the morning. The sun didn't rise in its usual way and my body lay motionless with only a dull pulse beating under a shroud of darkness. I look away to mask the secrets that are somewhat hidden behind my eyes. I tread quietly but my shadow falls too loudly, too suddenly and disturbs the peace. I have swallowed my own voice. Noises flow by in tiny murmurs, sounds that were once words but misplaced their significance somewhere along the way. Our roads merge and diverge without warning and without reason, while our minds wind their way through the unknown.

Even though my eyes are closing, my fingers still itch to write. The blood of my ancestors ripples through me and I write by the light of their departed stars. Their light flickers over the places that I cover up with solid smiles and murky reasoning, but with open arms and good intentions, I make my way across these deep and uncharted waters, because....well, because that is all I can do.

I draw a blank as to when or how I got to this place, but 'why', well I taste the 'why' as if it were a bee stinging my tongue. The fathers in my life are disappearing and without a choice, I must change gears. I embrace the change so my heart and my mind do not need to go into overdrive. I can sail smoothly, I can slow down, I can go where the wind takes me without that sickening fear that I am going to a place I shouldn't. I can push all those burnt bridges from my memory and today the world doesn't need to be on fire.

I need to breathe again. I need to be again. Stand my ground and swim the sea again. Learn to walk again, maybe even love again....... Lungs full of air and wanting to care again. Let the days lead us kindly to another, let the sun stain our faces and let our minds unearth a stillness that has never been touched.

Monique Potter
Australia

Maelstrom

I'm fighting my thoughts, fighting to breath,
Fighting to find myself buried under BPD.
This life is a labyrinth, just one big trick.
When you see a way out, the walls quickly shift.

As people got older they left me behind.
They realized they didn't have to put up with my kind.
They realized there is easier love to be found,
Where partners don't scream like a 3 year old and lay on the ground.

I used to know who I was – sensitive and angry, so what.
Now those are just symptoms. From the game of life I've been cut.
I'm the characteristics of my diagnosis, all 9 out of 9.
I'm tired. I'm happy. I'm scared. I'm fine.

But who am I now? I feel lost in the crowd.
According to society my chaotic emotions aren't allowed
I panic, I plead, "Can somebody help me please?!"
I'm losing myself; I'm down on my knees.

Can I re-write my own story into something worth living?
Will I ever escape from the memories, they're so unforgiving.
It's an earie feeling when you are able to reflect
On the moment in time you almost stole your own breath

Krista Simpson
Canda

Survival of the Fittest

Overwhelming sadness, it's here again
Depression; acting like a dear old friend
"Oh how I've missed you! Let me stay for a while"
I know the drill, head down, eyes blank, no smile
Reasons to feel happy elude me, my mind is clouded
I feel so hopeless, misery shrouded
I fear the worst; that I'm stumbling backwards
Disappointment rises to the surface; then something odd occurs
Disappointment turns to anger, anger to hatred
But I'm not angry at myself, I am elevated
This time I knock the monster off its feet, I stand overhead
"I'll make you pay for your deceit! I didn't forget the hateful things you said
You told me I had no future, I was nothing, just a waste of space
I bet you didn't think I'd rise above, staring down at your cowardly face
Now who's afraid of disappearing? It isn't me!
For I am on my way to victory
That's right, you parasitic thief!
You will not steal my hope and replace it with disbelief!
Because I've ripped your claws out of my head
I think the world would be a better place if you were dead!
Don't look so betrayed; don't look so stunned
It's survival of the fittest, and I have finally won!
Now you're fading away, returning to the place from which you came
You're not welcome here; I hope I never see you again"

Shawnna Hastings-Downey
Canada

Bittersweet

It's like ice in here though my skin is on fire. It's the first day of spring. The end of something and the beginning of something. My head has been opened up once again and all the sadness I had put to bed begins to stir. Perhaps if I stay here without looking it will go away. I strain to hear your voice above all the noise. I try and stay as close as I can to the edges so there's something to steady me when I slip. My words are dull and they lack any inspiration. My sentences are puddles of grey paste. Stow me away upon your highest shelf and put a trip wire at my feet. If I stay very still, I will no longer picture the faces and small voices echoing across miles of ocean. Those faces have haunted my dreams for too many nights. I will no longer have the need to be a better person, a better daughter, a better sister, a better friend. Guilt will not engulf me when I dream of rotting in a watery grave. No one will be left behind and I will no longer be troubled by the outside. All will be still as I let the dust settle over my porcelain form. My eyes of glass will see nothing and a pink smile will be neatly painted over my face. How very bittersweet...

Monique Potter
Australia

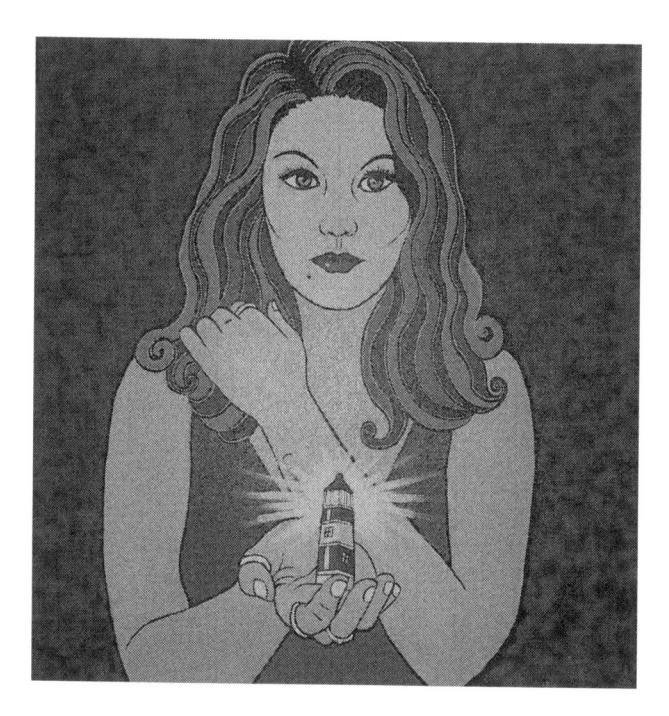

Proof of Light 2

Saadah Kent
Australia

Precariousness means walking on the tightrope and waiting for the fall and, for someone, keeping the balance tastes like an adventure. The feeling that you have to take advantage, that you can only devour - used as you are to fasting, as if you had to stock up before a long famine - prepares the moment of the surrender: daydreamed, foreseen, unavoidable.
Changes, for most people, are sceneries gradually shifting, to which you slowly get used. They are scenes fading from black to white, going through a wide range of colours to perceive, live, study; colours in which you can dive, to which you can get used slowly. For me, this is more and more rare. The change in the scenery appears to me complete already, all of a sudden, as if everything had happened without me knowing it, overnight, while I was asleep. I wake up and it's all there, ready made. The whole thing falls down on me.
Just only a conversation, a word, a gesture, and everything is suddenly and completely different.
It shakes me.
It influences my mood, my perception of myself and of the outer world, it "changes the structure of the rooms".
I'm the leaf in the wind as usual; I've got no roots. I'm the empty shell; how can I possibly be so evanescent? I've got no skin. I lack a layer. I'm flawed.
Take care of me. Can't you see I don't work well, I'm broken?
Hold me strong.
I'm endowed with a strong inclination to drama.
When things go wrong, I'm not able to contain the injury and take all the good that can still be taken. No. I go on digging until my nails and fingertips hurt.
A bit of bread, a slice of bread, half a kilogram of bread, a package of biscuits.
A detail out of place, an uncomfortable mattress, a word in the wrong moment, a sleepless night.
I really can't keep my balance, weigh my reactions, think about tomorrow instead of sobering my anger right now.

Moments of different lives succeed in the same day. Different persons, different bodies, as nothing had ever been before the terrible moment I'm living now. I try to give a meaning to this all, but there's no meaning. One year, two years, ten years... everything could be done in one moment. I recover, then a moment of carelessness is enough and I fall back again. Swollen tummy, headache, 5 o'clock in the morning, chocolate...

It can't be Penelope's shroud forever. It is. Living with this thing means accepting that there will be a few nice moments - spoiled by the anxiety that you must take advantage of them - and many horrible moments when everything will seem impossible to me. I'll wait for my fifteen minutes of glory and then down again. And I'll already know what's in store for me. But I'll go on hoping that someday everything will come to an end. And hope is the greatest of evils, the worst possible one. The one that keeps me, that holds me still, the one that should never be there.

Eleonora Nappi
Italy

Life has never been easy, it is a complicated world. Many would say that it is for everyone. Maybe it is. However living in my head is like living in a volcano, never know when or how it is going to erupt. I have tried everything thrown at me, yet nothing quite seems to work. Every day since I was 13 or so I have wished for a magic wand to fix it all. It has never come; I am beginning to think that maybe the wand is me, maybe I can fix it. However this small light is only there every few days coming and going as the volcano comes and goes. It feels hard to believe yourself each day when your mind is telling you constantly you are better off not existing, I see every mistake I make and it feels like a bomb going off; which in turn only reinforces the messages in my mind. The messages that I am bad, that everyone hates me, that I shouldn't be here. There is a light, so for now I am holding on. Tomorrow I might be back at the bottom of the pit again, with no light, no hope and no chance of helping myself.

This is a difficult thing to go through every day, however people have told me I see things in other people that others don't. Maybe it is everything I have been through allows me to empathise with others; though I am not convinced it is worth the pain I experience.

Amy Jennings
UK

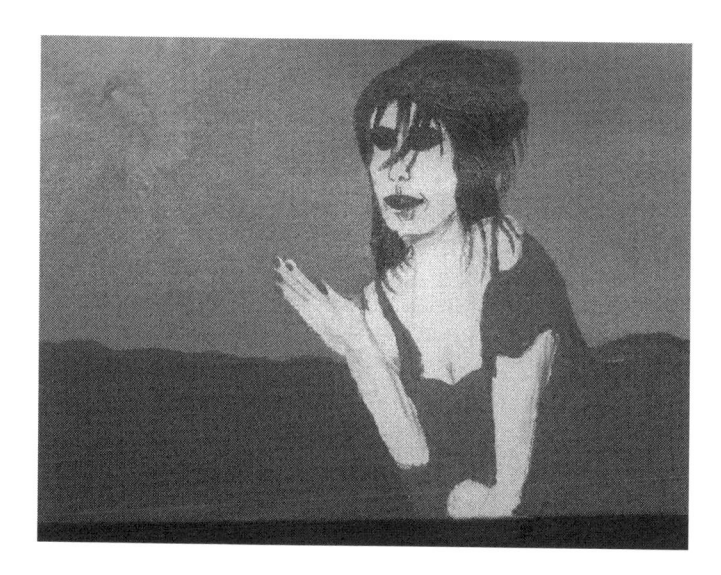

Untitled

Tee Taylor
UK

The Chance to Save a Life

If you had the chance to save someone, would you take it?
Could you deal with the pressure, could you really take it?
What if they were someone you knew, someone you were very close to?
Someone who's tired of trying because no matter what they do, their world is still bitterly blue
Crumbling, bland and bleak
Someone waving a white flag, admitting defeat
Someone who had hopes, someone who had dreams
Someone who is giving into the internal screams
Someone who feels they could not reach their full potential
Someone caught in the downpour while the rain is torrential
Would you be able to show them the way?
Make them truly believe that things will get better someday?
Would you be able to show them how to dance in the rain?
Show them how to better themselves through pain?
Would you be able to console?
Console the wreckage that is their heart, mind and soul?
Could you save them before it's too late?
Before they plan their greatest escape?
Could you make them see?
That they can be much stronger than misery?
I wonder; could you really put yourself in their shoes?
It's all up to me now; will they win or will they lose?
Because I am the person in question
Lost hope, lost direction
Do I have the strength to guide myself through?
Do I have the strength to show myself what to do?
Can I keep the self-destruction at bay?
My confidence is failing; I don't know if I have the strength to save myself today…
Do I really have the fight?
There's a tiny voice inside that whispers "I want to save a life…"

Shawnna Hastings-Downey
Canada

Amidst the binds of an unjust world
This tortured soul withers away
A dim moonlight cast
Thick fog washes through
Realisations of nightmares past
Hopes and terrors of the future
Rain smashes down to flood the path
Trails to be blazed, snuffed out
Dreams crashed upon the shore
As bashed by rocks amongst the waves
Tears are bled as the world crumbles
Torn apart on the edge of a shine
Pulsing rage blurs the lines
Pounding anger loses the boundaries
Twisted facts, breathe life
Stricken and condemned
Alone and broken down
Thrown aside and torn asunder
Left to drown in the deep
A beckoned call from broken pieces
Shards of hell under foot
Castle or cage depends on the view
The glare of escape, calling out
The thin line between relief and despair.

Rob Hernfield
Australia

"Mother" is the label of a God; not of thy God; written on the faces and spoken from the lips of all children. No concept of time.
The cry of a child comes first and will stay until death. It's not weakness but simply a prayer from the heart that beats faster. In that moment, a cry can turn to laughter with the power of affection; it may be very brief like that of a butterfly fluttering, splashing colours of confidence, yet can be turned into fear with that of rejection from the creator of their only world, they carry the fear with them until their last breath. Regretting the things they were too afraid to achieve. Because when you're in all forms of pain, the person you call to is your mother, in the name that became their God. To find clarity and peace;
"Please, God, help me"

Jessica Murray
Australia

Living in the darkness for so many years the moment of acceptance and self-learning has shown me a small light and given me hope that recovery is possible. To feel mentally healthy is a breath of fresh air.

JJ Harvey
UK

Darker Days

All that was tangible a few days ago has slipped like ashes through my finger tips. The faces and the names have disappeared and the sounds I heard as the sun rose and set each day have faded away and all I am left with is the dull thud of a giant heart that has nothing left to give. I write and I write until my finger tips are stained with ink from the moments where I have paused to think. I'm sitting under a palm watching my family in the water. I hang on tight like a torn appendage and I feel more alone than ever. I can't remember the moment when I stopped caring but I do remember the moment I knew that people's words were really just words. Meaningless words. No one says what they mean anymore. Perhaps like the words I'm writing, floating about in the Sydney sky. You may say that I'm not alone ten thousand times over but only I can make that call. I get tired of helping myself. I get tired of the days when my incompatibility with the rest of the world glares at the kind eyes of strangers. I get tired of laying heavy drapes over the same people's shoulders. My reasons for being here may not be the right ones but at least I can put some hearts at ease. I'm here. It doesn't matter to me. But I'm here. These are my darker days.

Monique Potter
Australia

BPD - GIFT OR CURSE:

Wow! I've just had a major epiphany!
I'm watching a TV show called Sense8. I don't want to give anything away but let's say the main characters in this show are in touch with their emotions. A bit of an understatement lol. There's one character that is guiding these other characters through their experience of feeling so deeply. One of the other characters asks this character: "Are we human?". His reply: "What is human? An ability to reason? To imagine? To love? To grieve? If so we are more human than any human will ever be."

I just thought to myself what a perfect description of BPD. We are more human than any other human on the face of the earth, and humanity has always had a positive connotation. Perhaps that's something to be proud of? Perhaps this is a gift rather than a curse? Maybe it just means that we have more of a moral responsibility than others? More of a social conscience? Maybe it means that we have the potential for greatness, the potential to change the world?

It made me ponder

Tania Neilson
Australia

I recently decided that I'm done hiding from my illness and that I actually want to get on with life, get my job back, get my friends back and just really really try to start life normally again.

But it really isn't that simple is it, not when you make all the plans to go ahead and do these things and all of a sudden you feel frightened and start thinking of the what if's, what if people ask questions about where I have been, what if I have another major break down in the middle of the street, what if just what if.

Being diagnosed with BPD really sets you back, I'm not going to lie. My job was affected by it and a lot of friendships I did have. I became so reclusive because all of a sudden I just simply could not trust anyone, I couldn't face the reality of the fact that I had been fighting for so long to beat the mental illness I was originally diagnosed with just for everything to fall apart around me and get diagnosed with another mental illness. No matter how many times I try and get on with things it is simply just not happening. Because once you recluse yourself so much into a world were you don't have to answer to anyone of how you're feeling or why you're not participating with outings with friends, you lose touch and that's when you start to realise months down the line that does it really get better from here. How much longer am I going to have to fight? Will I ever get my life back on track.

Charlotte Sharples
England

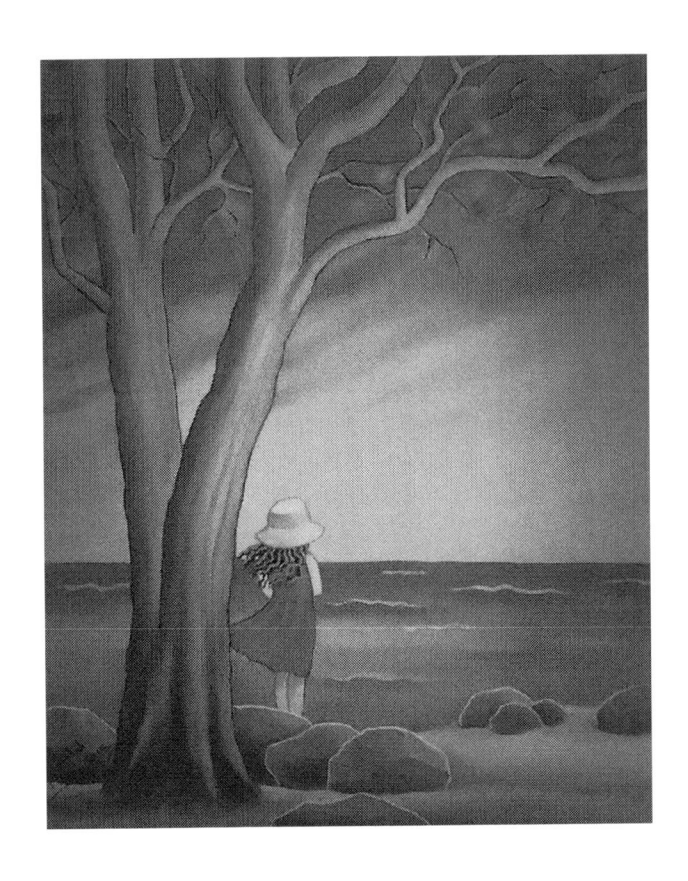

Finding My Feet

Saadah Kent
Australia

T'was not I

Remember it was you who started this with your hello
T'was not I

Remember it was you who was always planning for our future
T'was not I

Remember it was you who said you're life was much better with me
T'was not I

Remember it was you who said I love you first
T'was not I

Remember it was you who brought me into your world
T'was not I

Remember it was you who set us down this path
T'was not I

Remember it was you who got scared
T'was not I

Remember it was your lies that caused us to fail
T'was not mine

Remember it was you that began this pain
T'was not I

Remember it was you who gave up on me
T'was not I

Remember it was you who walked away
T'was not I

In the end it t'was I who will be left to remember
For in the end
It t'was I who saw it

When the time came to change it t'was you who said
Sorry,

T'was not you
Nor t'was it I?

Within this illusion
Within my own lie
I can no longer see you
I can only see I

Once to be life long friends
Pushed too far
Now left only to wonder
How it all went so wrong

I had faith hope and love
For the person I created
But the person I created
He's not who you are
Toady I am left to understand all along
It T'was I.

Rachel Coen
USA

VI.

Recovery

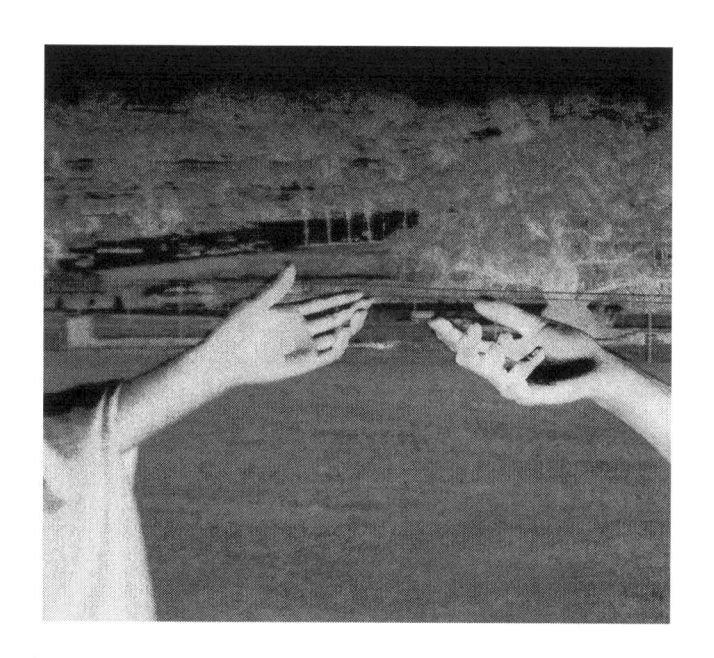

Helping Hand

Melanie Carrillo
USA

I know that I'm broken, I've accepted that now,
I long to be fixed, but I don't know how,
Years of fighting, looking for clues,
A cure, magic pills, no longer the blues.

Relationships formed, relationships ended,
Friendships I treasured that can't ever be mended,
Dreams that I had, dreams never achieved,
Praying for moments I could feel reprieved.

Feeling alone in the busiest of crowd,
Longing to feel I could make someone proud,
Hiding the pain behind a laugh or a smile,
To know happy again, it could be a while.

I push people away, I crave their return,
Closeness means pain, this I did learn,
So I wander along, left out just to roam,
I want to belong, be part of a home.

Yet this is my lot, it's just how I am,
I hold back the tears, I've built up a dam,
I know that tomorrow I may wake up happy,
Loving my life, all giddy and yappy.

These are the days I treasure the most,
When my quirky self is the perfect host,
I am determined again, ambitious and strong,
Feel that I, will never do wrong.

I know that my illness doesn't define me,
Remembering I am Katie is always the key,
To continue my life as best as can be,
I will learn to love life and live life with my bpd.

Katie Acton
England

Group Therapy:

The wings of fire swoop down from the sky

Little grains of silica flow from the flaming claws

Forming the hourglass which frames the free falling escapees

Down and around the circumference of time.

The lost ones, who search for their souls

Unable to find the entrance or is it exit

To the water

To emerge whole

To extinguish the pain from which they came.

Karine Stampe
Canada

I've spent the last 14 years wishing I was dead because of bpd. It's a curse. It isn't attention seeking. It's soul destroying. Incredibly painful. It's like a cancer. It eats away at and ruins all that is good about a person. It's a daily fight to keep things in perspective. It's a living hell. It makes you wish you hadn't been born. It's not depression, it's worse than depression because you keep getting your life back, you get so much hope, then you self sabotage everything. It's an evil condition. Those of us who work at trying to understand it and therapy to change.... it's soooo hard

Anonymous
UK

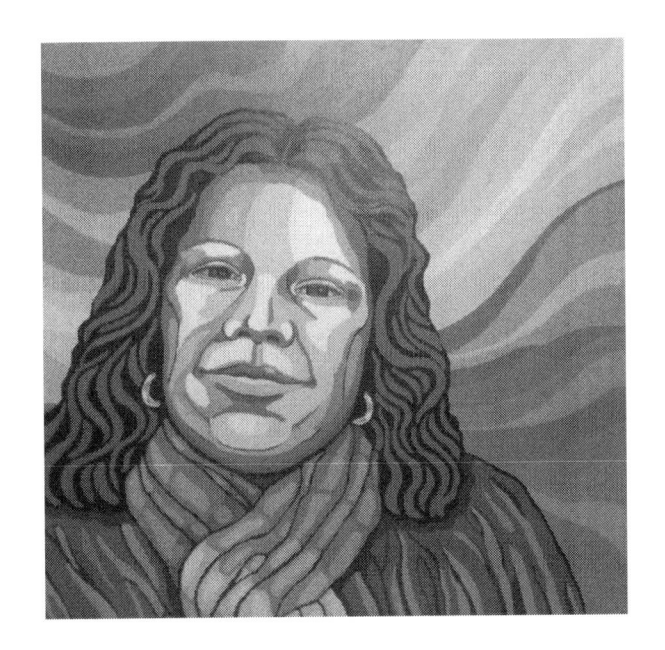

Self Portrait - Better Days

Saadah Kent
Australia

Real Families Facing Real Crisis:

I forced myself to read the entire denial yesterday.

It was 12 pages of drivel, talking about all these things I had neither heard nor seen. The judge asserted several times I was lying and playing the system. He placed most weight on the original (student) Psych who was very difficult and ended up having me go to someone else. I saw him 2x.

Much of it felt personal. He spent an entire page explaining why my diagnosing therapists' letter was not used and in his words "discarded." He stated that only a Dr (Per the law or his reading of it) can be given weight when determining disability. He pointed out I had seen 3 therapists (1st one moved, 2nd one was more nuts than me and I have seen Jeff since Aug. but they only had my records through Sept. 5th -Hearing was Oct 29th)

He stated that to qualify for disability for my back I had to be in treatment and being monitored by a Physician. He chose not to weigh in or acknowledge that I had, through no fault of my own, been without insurance since Sept. 1st. So I can't see the back and Ortho Doctor's.

The irony should be somewhat evident. Take away my insurance then deny me disability because I have no insurance.

Here is the cost to my family. We would have qualified for insurance through disability (Medicare and in KS [surprisingly] auto puts Medicaid secondary) back pay of around $25,000+ net (after taxes/attorney) $2103/month (our expenses are around $2200/month)

We have $1.97 in checking. We have rent paid for Dec then we will be facing shutoffs on utilities. My wife has no family to speak of, my father turns 70 and is going on a fixed income. In addition, because of my Mother's stroke, Dad is unable to gift money above a certain amount ($500?) so it has to be in the form of a loan. Which we are about $15,000 in debt to him.

This is pretty devastating to us. While those that have followed my story here know that I lost all confidence in this process a long time ago. I wasn't "banking" on winning in spite of an attorney (Till the hearing) telling me we had a great chance, I definitely meet the conditions.

I have no idea what I will do. I don't even know what I can physically do. My back and hip have deteriorated. The MRI's 2 years apart showed significant changes and we are now a year later. For my part.. I should have pushed more on the back. I was so focused on avoiding surgery and/or pain meds that I may have inadvertently under emphasized those issues.

I should have played the game. Trips to the ER, perhaps a weekend away on a psych hold. He never referenced my 2 sessions where we did talk about In Patient as in early May I started crashing hard. I wasn't sleeping and my emotions were so raw....

I really hope if people read this they refrain from saying "It will be ok." That very much diminishes my situation and if we are going to be honest on here then we need to accept that sometimes it really is bad. There really are not easy answers. Real people feel the pain of stigma and decisions and judges, etc....

This is my life, not just a "story." My 6 and 12 year old girls are real, they breathe, eat and poop and everything. (sorry needed some humor)

I am aware that all I can do is hope my insurance is reinstated. Go back to surgery, ortho and pain Dr. There comes a point though where I have to feed my family.

And people wonder why I don't want to be in the "present."

Michael Johnson
USA

I hate the diagnosis. I think people react as though there is a wretched wild animal in the room that cannot be controlled or trusted. I have expressed healthy, legitimate thoughts and feelings, and been told I am being irrational due to mental illness. My ex husband was very abusive, and when I started to seek help, he told people I was crazy and was making things up because I was "mentally ill". I also had a psychiatrist for a while who was extremely sexual inappropriate and crossed boundaries. I was afraid to tell anyone because I figured he'd deny it and call me crazy and manipulative too. And I was even more afraid that people would believe him over me. My friend, a social worker, who also has bpd, told me that bpd is essentially a label of "bad behaviour" and that professionals generally have little patience in dealing with us. I have experienced this on several occasions. I have worked with some very good, compassionate and caring professionals too, but the stigma of the "bpd" label really bothers me. I think it is the worst diagnosis.

Anonymous

I feel like now that my immediate crisis is over everyone around me is ready to say, "build a bridge and get over it", and I'm trying to, but unfortunately my bridge building kit came with Ikea instructions and is made of shoddy materials that break under any pressure. Build a bridge and get over it, yeah that's my goal, but I need to get the proper material and instructions first then I can make it across and out of this mess.

Anonymous

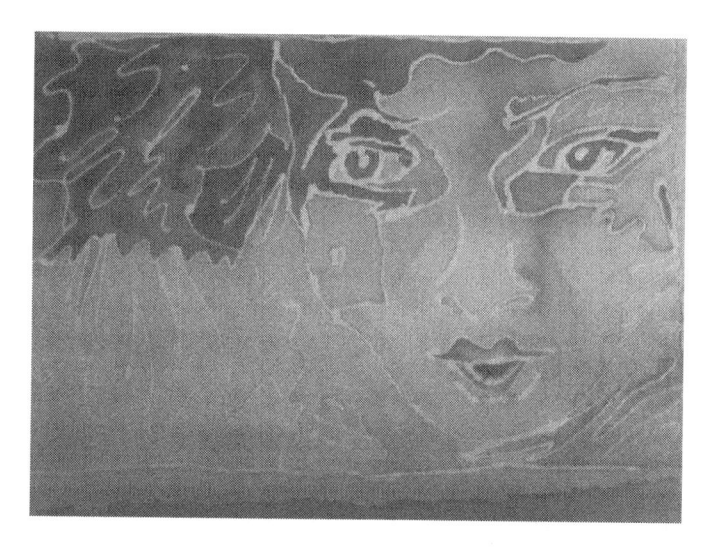

Untitled

Tee Taylor
UK

Breaking Free Within the Disorder

It consumes me. It's constant. And it's unrelenting. I hold such resentment toward my disorder, particularly for the deepest and darkest 2 ½ years of my life. During that time it felt like my life stopped. And in a way it did. It became completely different. My daily goal was to stay alive. When I crossed some imaginary line between struggling and recovery and my life felt like it started again I would look in the mirror (and still do daily) and see someone who had aged so much. I look old, warn, sad, drained. I look like I was tested. And I was. And I won. But winning has never been enough to remove the resentment towards BPD for taking those years of my life and making the years following the dark period so difficult. I hated what I saw in the mirror and often still do. I am still angry and bitter for the loss of those years. I am still angry and bitter for how those years changed me (yes some has been good, but most has been challenging and difficult). Sometimes I miss who I was before the diagnosis. Even though I sometimes struggled when I was younger, it seems that along with the labels comes knowledge and awareness that is such a double edged sword.

My first hospital bracelet says I was 32 and this year I will be turning 37. Although over 2 years has gone by since those dark times faded, things never went back to the easy carefree way they were before. I was a fairly regular person – happy but quiet, and sometimes angry, anxious, or sad. But I never owed anyone an explanation for it, I never had to take medication for it, and I never had to go to therapy for it. Everything is different now. Everything is harder. Every situation is harder. Every conversation is harder. Every moment is harder.

One of the hardest parts about recovery has been the fear of failure. After I was diagnosed with BPD I was constantly "falling down". It was easier in the beginning because nobody expected anything significant from me. I just had to stay alive and on a good day I had to get off the couch. But now that I have been in recovery for about two years my fear of failure has magnified. Nobody used to notice when I fell down because I fell down constantly. As I started to improve I noticed that every little failure would place a spotlight on me. Even if I was just having an off day those close to me would ask if something bad happened or if I had hurt myself (even if the last time had been months and eventually years behind me). Even though the dark times had ended I was still living in the most ominous shadow.

I have been buried alive by my own thoughts, by the symptoms, and even by the act of getting better. I could never have anticipated that one of the most challenging parts of this journey would be the pain and anguish associated with a greater awareness of my disorder, my thoughts and my behaviours. I constantly have a panel of critics inside my head who analyze everything I do and don't do, everything I say and don't say, everything I feel and don't feel and shouldn't feel. I am constantly on stage expected to present my best self, better than yesterday and certainly better than a year ago, never mind two. My head is so full of information – therapy, tools, "handy" acronyms, research articles, and tips from psychiatrists, family and the odd Facebook post. I feel like everyone is watching, not from a typical BPD sense of being judged, but from the sense that they are waiting for me to slip, watching in fear. I am under the most intense scrutiny, but not from others, from myself. I am all too cautious as I navigate my recovery.

They say I have far surpassed the expectations of therapists in terms of recovery from BPD. But why should those with BPD only aspire to just get off the couch, hold a job and sustain a relationship? I want to live life, travel, develop my career and thrive in a relationship so I can grow old with someone special who doesn't just put up with me. Why should merely managing symptoms be good enough? Good enough has never been good enough for me. Even though I struggle every day, I did get off the couch and even climbed mountains, I have advanced quickly in my career and my sights are set high, and I am in a healthy relationship with someone who encourages me to be the best I can be. And I still want to do more and be more. Despite the challenges and resentment and the person I sometimes see in the mirror, I no longer just believe, but I know that I will be free.

Krista Simpson
Canada

I'd like to scrap the BPD label altogether. When I was diagnosed 10 years ago the psychiatrist wrote 'Borderline personality (disorder)' on a piece of paper, warned me to be careful who I told or how I used that label, and said I was best off trying self-help as many people believed it to be incurable. 10 years on I'm still coming to grips with it, and my god, DBT is not only helpful, it's common sense! Validation is the most essential thing for me: my pain is real, and even if it seems incomprehensible, it can in fact be explained to people patient enough to listen. We need to stop pathologising emotional sensitivity. In fact it's the lack of empathy and fellow-feeling in our culture that is pathological. "It is no measure of health to be well adjusted to a profoundly sick society".

Libby Boyd
Thailand

There is the truth, then there are lies, and our life, well, it lays somewhere in between.

Anonymous

Unfortunately depression is tricky. Sometimes it's chronic, sometimes it's situational. Hell, sometimes it's not even depression, but a personality disorder that manifests similar symptoms. At the end of the day, the management of all of it is the same, though.

Depression may prevent *some* of these tasks, but as a chronic sufferer myself, I have found that if I give myself a break and simply do as much as I can, one thing at a time, every day, it gets easier. And some days it's REALLY HARD and I'm angry every second about having to do any of it, but I fight through it and do it anyway. Some days all I manage is feeding myself or drinking water and the rest of it is spent in bed crying or sleeping. But I still accomplished eating and hydrating.

We MUST exaggerate and make a big deal out of the successes, as our emotional responses are hardwired to do the opposite and we gotta take the lead on rerouting them. It can be done with a shit load of time, consistency, and patience with yourself. But each and every one of us are worth it.

Christine Jones
USA

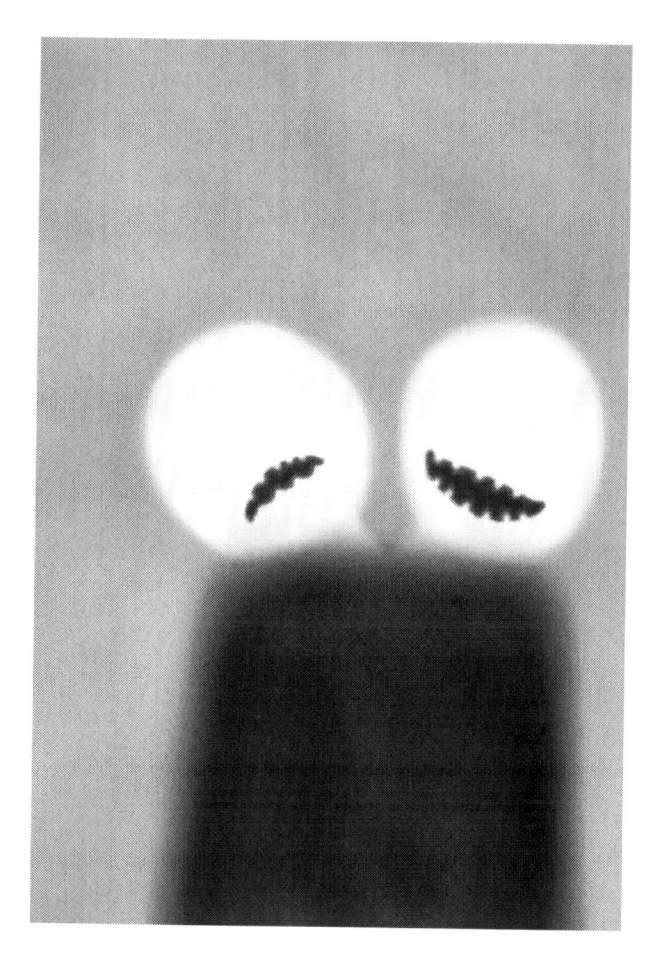

Two Sides

Cody White
Australia

"Lonely Road"

I wake up and tell myself... this will be the day... the day I can get up and go make something of myself. The day I'll stop being afraid... But it's never the day. The time is never right. Is it me who's never right? I search inside myself for some sort of strength to push myself... to keep crawling when I can't walk... so that I can learn to walk and learn to run... and from there learn to jump and from there learn to fly.

What do you do when you know deep down you're meant to soar? But you can't quite find your wings... they feel so clipped and sometimes I feel so crippled from doing anything at all. One day at a time they all say. Do they know that... just one day feels like a lifetime? That I feel like I am pulling myself inside out as I continue to try to pull myself... out of myself. Do they know that this is how it feels every second I breathe and that no degree... and no amount of intelligence can change this emotional block... this mental strain?

I'm a Credential Peer Support Specialist and still barely unable to leave my home. I've had the certification for 2 months. I am still so afraid to work. To be around people terrifies me. Where is the sense? Where is the trust? Do any of them ever truly know how we all struggle to find our way? That we have anxiety about anxiety, searching to find some type of normalcy in hopes to fit in... somewhere... anywhere.

We know... and we band together in this fight. And we will keep on fighting and supporting each other through it. They can't take that away from us. And they'll never have our courage. They'll never know how much we struggle. And how much we wish they would stand beside us, instead of against us. We just need someone to be there, and stay there. Because everyone leaves us, on this lonely road.

Marry Whitaker
USA

Let It Be Known

Let it be known, let it be told
That I have never dealt with anything quite as intricate as my own soul
So many pieces, pieces of me
So many feelings of varying degrees, varying intensities
I used to feel so broken, so shattered, outworn
Imperfect, improper, forlorn
Eventually I realized what I needed was perspective
And that changing negative beliefs may be effective
Instead of comparing myself to what once was
I began to look at the here and now, that is because
I've already grieved for my former self, many times I have mourned
Can't afford to drown in guilt, or feel so utterly torn
I then decided to let go of some things I cannot change;
To look at things from a different angle; to completely rearrange
Live in the present moment
To become more aware, more focused
Challenge the way I perceive myself
My life, self-worth, and health
Tried to see the good in things
Put down the tape, the glue, the strings
Could these pieces, turn out to be something beautiful?
If they can, I'm sure such beauty would be indisputable
All of my pieces, so colourful and jagged
Are not reasons to judge myself harshly or feel bad
For there is no shame in being me
Full of surprise and inconsistency
Like a kaleidoscope, I am ever changing, and the shifts, well they shed light

I'm not damaged, I'm a work in progress, these
pieces represent freedom, not a sorrowful
plight
And when I look at myself, when I stare very
hard
I begin to see little splinters and shards
Things that over time did not change
Maybe my essence in fact, remained the same
Maybe I didn't lose myself in the pitfall
Maybe, just maybe, I'm still a decent person
after all

Shawnna Hastings-Downey
Canada

The Beast Won't Break Me

I polish all the tools and skills I am armed with, knowing that the feelings are only visitors. They come and go, even on days where I feel like they've made themselves at home and seem ready to move in. 'They are only here for a short stay' I whisper into my pillow. Never have anyone tell you your feelings aren't real. They are as real as the sun rises every morning. Sometimes I am sad for no reason at all, but feeling sad doesn't mean we will never be happy. Feelings are only feelings. Allow yourself to feel them. I am at peace with this cloak I have draped over my shoulders. I do not question its existence because I could search every corner of the universe and still be no closer to finding an answer. I don't need an answer but I do need a solution. I have spent many years learning how to tame the beast inside me. Sometimes it's just the tiniest of actions or the whisper of words and all of a sudden I've grabbed onto something, a speck of something and before I know it, I can feel it crawl beneath my skin.

How you say a word, what you put before or after it can make the sentence choke me or merely pass me by. We have to remind ourselves that we don't see things as they are. We see them as we are. Sometimes the words cut into my flesh that is already missing several layers of skin. I bleed, but the bleeding stops. And the beauty is, I know that it stops. I cry a thousand tears with the pain of an army of sorrows, but the tears stop. And the beauty is, I now know that they will stop. I can't stop the pain of a thousand knives but I am wise enough to know that the stabs become pin pricks and then a tingle and then they disappear. The more the tears are ignored, the longer they will stay. If you take the tears and acknowledge them, indulge them, though they feel insatiable, they will soon find another home.

Anais Nin once wrote:
'I despise my own hypersensitiveness, which requires so much reassurance. It is certainly abnormal to crave so much to be loved and understood.'

I read this and I smile because it is the truth, my truth, and so many other people's truths, and all I can do is laugh because the absurdity of our states of mind come to light, and I can only love them and laugh.

My feet are planted firmly on the ground but I accept the moments where I feel like the beast is breaking me, because I know it is just passing through. Just saying hello. A friend I love to hate.

Monique Potter
Australia

The answers are NOT in the bottom of a coffee cup,

Nor in the bottom of a whiskey glass,

They are NOT in the final piece of pie or the last spoonful of cake,

They are NOT at the end of a brisk walk, or looking out to sea,

They are NOT in the words of our friends or lovers,

They are NOT at the end of a shopping spree or even in the church,

They are NOT in poetry or songs or books,

They are NOT in holidays or spontaneous daytrips,

They are NOT in therapy or spirituality,

They are NOT in sleeping or dreaming or driving,

They are NOT at home,

They are NOT in anything we can do or touch or see,

Yet we keep searching, hoping to find the answers, which may never come.
When you have searched high and low where else is their to go?
I have looked for the answers of which I don't even know the question.
In all the things I've seen, felt and experienced it's never there.
The result is NOT for eternal happiness,
Just for inner peace and a quiet mind, that is all I desire.
Nothing more.

Ann Font Vanrell
UK

I wish we didn't have to label ourselves, as sometimes we identify so much with the label that it becomes us in a lot of ways, and hampers us more than helps us. I understand the need, but I have had so many labels attached to me (11) and after awhile I finally found a therapist who said. "Discard all the labels and don't focus on any of them, this is just the way your brain adapted to keep you safe in an unsafe environment. Accept all parts of yourself, even (and especially) the ones you don't like, because they were all there for a reason, even if that reason no longer exists (being in a traumatic environment). Your behaviors and habits are all coping mechanisms induced by traumatic experiences.

Nancy Bearup
USA

I was diagnosed with BPD and type II bipolar two years ago after an attempted suicide. My wife left me after researching the diseases and deciding that I was never going to get better. I believed her for the longest time. Every day I woke up and instantly defeated myself. I told myself I was unlovable, that I was scum and that it would never get better.
Well, I'm getting better. It's a slow process but I finally live in a world that isn't rife with emotional triggers. It took 29 years to realize that I needed to do it for myself but here I am.

Nate Brown
USA

I stopped myself from giving a shit about what people thought of me, forgave myself, and my tormentors for my past, and radically accepted my situations as they arose.
You can have peace and calm, you just have to focus and learn to trust in yourself again,

BPD must be treated like an unpredictable leashed beast. Keep it in line, discipline it- and don't let it take control. Learn everything about it; what sets it off; when does it turn on you? ECT. Reign it in and own it. And also embrace it – for bpd is more common than you'd imagine – and you can spot it within other once you understand it.

It's everywhere.

Harry Oliver
New Zealand

When you have searched high and low where else is their to go?
I have looked for the answers of which I don't even know the question.
In all the things I've seen, felt and experienced it's never there.
The result is NOT for eternal happiness,
Just for inner peace and a quiet mind, that is all I desire.
Nothing more.

Ann Font Vanrell
UK

When I first got a diagnosis, I was so happy to finally have a path to recovery, to know that I could finally address it. Now, doctors are reluctant to help me with anything, not just mental health, but physical health issues as well, are just considered a manipulation and attention seeking ploy. I've never used drugs, but doctors tell me that they are hesitant to prescribe anything beyond antibiotics because of my "mental health history".

I've recently been told I was misdiagnosed, but the label is still there. They won't remove it."

Courtney Foal
Australia
Fighter and survivor

To live is to learn...to learn is to know...to know is to be in control.
KNOW your emotions, recognize them, experience them, and move on from them. Only then do you gain true control."

Jennifer Purvis
USA

MY TAKE ON BPD:

The way I think of my BPD is like a broken bone or a torn muscle. It may heal but there will be a tenderness there, a fragility beneath the surface, and if placed under stress could elicit a flare up. Damn I'm proud of that analogy! Lol. Sounds pretty good if I don't say so myself! Lol.

If we work on our mental health we build resilience and we become less vulnerable to taking one or one thousand steps back when going through tough patches in our lives.

I understand where you're coming from because I've felt the very same way oh countless times. My initial reaction is frustration but if you think about it, being reminded of how far you've come and what you've conquered is a bit of a gift.

Our minds are pretty amazing. A slight shift in the way we view something can change our whole world

Tania Neilson
Australia

Demons:

I wish I could tell everyone that I am doing better, on my way, etc....but I am afraid that is not the truth.

I vacillate between moments of intense searing pain and just a numb feeling. I have started to realize a few things about myself like- I really don't feel like I fit in. I spent my whole life trying to "fit in" to what I thought people wanted me to be and that was a miserable experience. If I focus on the present it's very painful and frankly feels pretty hopeless at times.

My therapist moved. We rarely communicated via e-mail or phone, but I would e-mail her occasionally. She was an integral part of my story, and she was the first therapist I have felt like I could tell her anything and she would understand. She exhibited incredible patience with me, she allowed me to proceed at my pace.

This also meant my daughter lost her therapist and that was really hard on her. We each had a visit with a new therapist and neither was really a fit. So we contacted the agency asking for 1 therapist, that was part of our attraction originally. It allows the therapist to give us insight as to how the other thinks, reacts, etc....They said to give them a week or two. It's important to feel safe, much like a pregnant mother needs to feel with their OB. Otherwise therapy is pointless.

To see the way the world affects my 12 year old is hard. Parents know this: I would gladly take every ounce of her pain so she could be happy. Nothing is harder than watching pain in the eyes of those you love. I've come to realize she is growing up (way too fast), her problems are real and need to be taken seriously.

Therefore it's easier to just tell folks I am "ok." Because if I answer differently it either spirals me downward or begs the inevitable question, "What's wrong." A very
well intentioned question, but very stigmatic to people with depression....as though we can control it or have an easy answer.

I have gained a better understanding about DBT, its pluses and minuses. I also have been able to figure out my resistance or struggle with it.

I've blogged at length
about individualized treatment plans, not presenting DBT as pass/fail,
and acknowledgment that it doesn't always work and that's
ok....without immediately jumping to the conclusion that there is something "wrong" with the person and that it can't be fixed.

For me, I think its pretty simple. I'll use a back pain analogy. Which I have a lot of. As I have gotten older and have documented issues with my back they finally quit preaching "Physical therapy" possibly at all but at least not until we had THE PAIN UNDER CONTROL

Same thing with BPD with an additional diagnosis of severe depression

I've spent my whole life sweeping these moments of pain under the rug, not dealing with them. Not accepting the totalitarianism of certain events and relationships. Let me be clear here...there is a difference between understanding your illness and managing it. I maintain that with this illness the pain of realization may outweigh some of the advantages.

So... I have seen about 8 therapists. 2 for a year (90 and 93) the rest 1 visit. Haven't been in therapy in 20 years and half my story has occurred during that time. I think its real simple here... I need therapy to heal the wounds, old and new. I need patience, kindness, understanding and believing in me, even when it doesn't look good at that moment.

What I don't need is someone with a preconceived notion. Someone that wants to set a time frame for my recovery and coping skills. Mostly just someone that understands I am in pain, even when I say I am not.

Michael Johnson
USA

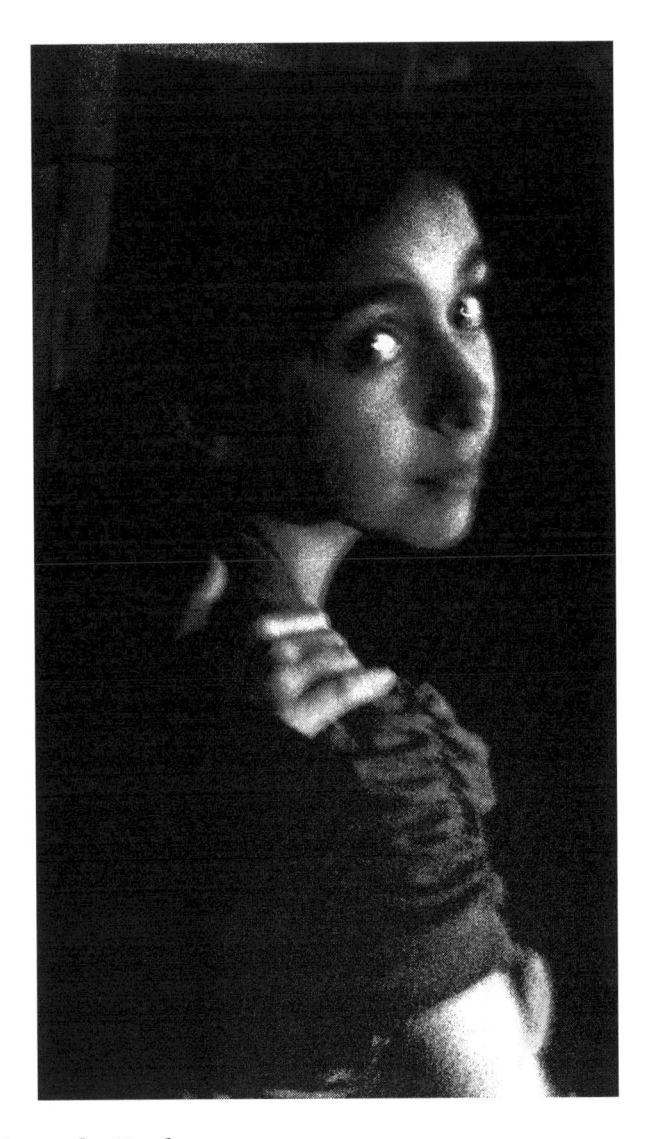

From the Darkness

Melanie Carrillo
USA

This morning, as I was lying in bed, I began thinking about all of the things people with BPD experience but don't talk about.

Things that aren't listed on the DSM like early wake, eating disturbances, hearing voices, feeling like there is someone in the room, disassociation, derealization and so on...

I know for me I never talked about them because I didn't know other people didn't experience these things too, and when I found out I was different I didn't want people to think I was more crazy than I am. Now I don't care. I talk about what I experience open and honestly. People need to know what you are going through in order to understand why you act the way you do.

I have found that most people who don't have bpd don't understand, but for those of us who do we find comfort in finding out others are like us. To know we aren't alone in our quirks, especially those we don't mention, makes the everyday battle a little less lonely

M.E.

I just wish everyone knew that what's seen as symptoms of our disorder now, is what saved us in the past..

It's not about being 'difficult' or 'dramatic'..

At least, not on purpose..

It's just..

What saved us..

A way of surviving, for so long, it became a part of us..

Ida Emilie Sommervold Vea
Norway

My truth and yours may or may not be the same, but the fact is as long as its truth to you, it IS truth. But remember this... Truth= perception...fact= reality."

Jennifer Purvis
USA

I wish people would HONESTLY understand that we don't try to be difficult... That we try so hard to be "normal" and some of us manage to pull that off well most of the time so if I am under a lot of stress and such and I slip up and show an odd behavior or impulse control then. It's because there is something major going on and it's out of my hands. You don't get mad when a diabetic has to eat or take a shot so please stop getting mad when I need to take a break or walk away to compose myself.

Laura Lee
USA

THANK YOU FOR MY PAIN:

It took me a hell of a long time to realise this; that pain is actually my gift. The best pieces I've ever written were because I have experienced pain. They were either the description of pain or they were inspiration that comes from pain, but nonetheless pain was a necessary presence. So today I say thank you for the pain because I believe that my suffering and endurance of pain gives me the ability to write; the good, the bad, the ugly, the most desperate and the most optimistic and hopeful. And that is my gift to the world. I hope you like it.

Tania Neilson
Australia

Saving Grace

I wrote this poem as a tribute to the person I hurt the most whilst being hospitalised and losing myself and my mind completely. Though, in my mind, I had treated her as badly as you could treat another human being, not for one second did she ever consider giving up on me. She was my saving grace. This is for her and all the other friends and family who have had to witness their loved ones going through what some of us can only describe as hell and not being able to stop the pain.

In this small patch of sunlight, I feel myself grow. I think of you often, and more than you know. I silently thank you for holding my hand, while I clung to a thread with my head in the sand.

I searched for some peace and I pleaded my case, while my spirit dissolved in this pitiful place. Meanwhile, I watched your heart in suspense, in me, you struggled to find any sense.

Wild eyed and raging, I ran and I fell. I landed face down in this sweet private hell. I tried to get up but the waves dragged me down, so I wandered the halls in a cold cotton gown.

I lost all my senses, my rights and my mind. My actions weren't measured, but still so unkind. I cannot erase, rewind or press pause, but I pray that you'll see that I'm not a lost cause.

I refuse to let go or give up on this fight, my knuckles translucent and holding on tight. The same grip you had on me, drowning at sea, even though you could recognise nothing in me.

I write this in silence; a shaking of hand. Free
falling from somewhere. Who knows where I'll
land. I do know for certain the sting of this
climb,
 but I'm taking it all one day at a time.

I hope that in time you forgive me my faults,
 my flaws and my shame and my thoughtless
assaults. I know you need time, some air and
some space,
 but never forget – you are my saving grace.

Monique Potter
Australia

The Beginning

Depression can render you mute: incapable of voicing your needs, because you don't know what it is that you need. It can worsen the trepidation of voicing your emotions, because all you know is sadness. It can cripple your ability to effectively express love because all you really fully understand is your hatred toward yourself.
Not only did I ignore it, I embraced it, like so many others. I found ways to push myself further and further into territory that, so far, has manifested itself as a sort of no-man's land: desolate, lonely, bleak, and unnavigable. I have found myself lost and defeated in this confusing landscape, and still I wander further and further into this monochromatic world. I don't enjoy the scenery, it's a scenery that stares back at you--but it is all I know. It's home.

I am currently receiving treatment for a variety of mental ailments. Certain disorders that are difficult to treat, and nearly impossible for others to tolerate. I've gained enough clarity through my infancy in treatment to ruminate, somewhat unkindly, upon the past and the chain of carelessness, self doubt, hypocrisy, arrogance, and manipulation that eventually convinced me to upturn a beautiful life with an absolutely beautiful person, culminating in various suicide attempts and months of aching for the ability to change the past.

I have somewhat anthropomorphized depression/anxiety into an entity that hung me from puppet strings and forced me to dance for it. In some ways I suppose it did, but only because I granted it that control. My struggles came from within, though I continuously projected them onto others in a desperate attempt to convince myself that I was fine--it was everyone else who was broken. I was unhappy with my marriage due to problems that berthed from my own mind. I placed the responsibility of my happiness upon my loving and loyal wife, and she bore it as well as any single human being could. Even after I told her about all of the twisted and awful things I had done.

Nate Brown
USA

The best we can hope for with BBD is to live with BPD traits, not active disease, and like diabetes this requires special doctors and a healthy life style. It's about knowing what makes us well, acknowledging what temps us to act out, and be in tune with our body and listen when it tells us what we need.

Livia Richard
USA

I've had enough of dreary days
I've got to be tough
I've got to find ways
To enjoy this life
The precious time given to me
I'll try with all of my might
To find peace and be happy
No more tears
No more sorrow
I'll conquer my fears
In hopes of a better tomorrow
So watch me succeed
Watch me grow
I'll find the strength to believe
This I know
One day, things will be better
I'll do a 180
And finally get my life together
Things will improve greatly
It will get better
Just wait and see!

Shawnna Hastings-Downey
Canada

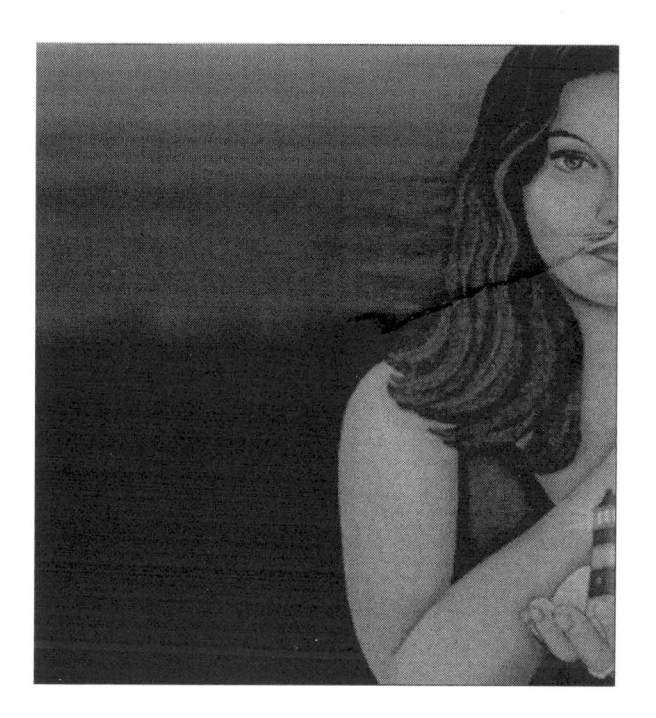

Proof of Light 4

Saadah Kent
Australia

I learned this easy oversimplification: illnesses are defenses; they are weapons, control, an anaesthetic. To me, life is feeling it all without filters. It's like a falling avalanche. From armor to absence of skin. Both bring a rainfall of tears, and yet they are so different that trying to tell them apart is a total waste of words.

To me, taking care of myself is the hardest task ever. At every occasion, at every distraction or light gesture, the temptation to fall is always strong. I constantly have to bring myself back to reality, tap myself on the shoulder, rationalize the situation and negotiate. Sometimes I feel like sliding until I can't reach myself anymore, but I know I can't afford that any longer.

I wish somebody was there to protect me, to limit the damages, to help me stay alive and never go back, to build and not cover. An assistant, an existential guide, someone who could protect me from myself in favor of life, someone who could tie me to him forbidding me to escape.

Healing is ceasing to resist. It's surrendering, knowing when to ask for help with easy and clear words, giving myself up to nourishment and trust. It is knowing how to say, "I need this" and to accept it and receive it. It is ceasing to continually doubt my instincts; it is learning how to recognize my own needs and meet them. It is capability of saying, "I beg you, it's now time for you to guide me and for me to rest."
And with every little step, here comes some relief, a muscle relaxing, a little piece of sky lightning up, a little bit of fluidity in my thoughts.

Healing is knowing how to pray. But you can't pray if you don't learn how to exist first; if you don't know how to accept that you are here to occupy space and to make noise, if you don't know how to recognize your worth.

Healing is creating sense out of nothingness, even fixing nothingness. Something is always going to rise from nothing. Madness fills the void. Hunger fills the void. Neurosis fills the void. Writing fills the void. Life itself fills the void. The void can be filled in two ways: with life or with illness. But it can never stay the same. I want to live. I want to write that down so it can be impressed somewhere, so that my thoughts can be read, so it will be clear, even when I feel like dying, that a part of me wanted to live. I want to live, I don't want this illness.

Eleonora Nappi
Italy
Translated by Ombretta Di Dio

Index of Authors

A

Acton, Katie 236

Anonymous 2, 18, 127, 144, 148, 237, 242, 247

Ayers, Loretta 161-171

B

Bearup, Nancy 128, 257

Bernardo, Nicole 77

Betty, Jody 133-135, 182-183

Boyd, Libby 22-23, 247

Bridges, Clara 53-58
Extract taken from "Waiting to fall – BPD and obsessive attachments" published from the blog http://lifeinabind.com/ on 21 July 2014

Broderick, Naomi Mercedes 138

Brown, Nate 96-98, 109-110, 140-142, 257, 270-271

C

Carrillo, Melanie 39, 64-65, 69, 83, 111, 139, 235, 264

Celeste, Erin 63

Chambers, Nate 104-105

Chaudhuri, Arundhati 152-154

Chloe 74

Cline-Saia, Allison 74

Clothier, Colleen 34

Coen, Rachel 99, 231-232

Cornall, Courtney 44

Cradick, Hannah 63

D

Delissa 143

DuPlessis, Freda 10, 82

E - G

Elizabeth, Dion 187

Figiel, Hayley 45

Foal, Courtney 75, 259

George, Jennifer 1, 6-7, 17, 67, 72

H

H., Scott 159-163

Harrington, Kevin 73, 143

Harvey, JJ 226

Hastings-Downey, Shawnna 24, 46, 68, 117, 172, 181, 217, 224, 252-253
Exceperts from Emotive:
Living with Borderline Personality Disorder
And
Metamorphosis:
My Journey through Dialectical Behaviour Therapy

Heaney, Stacey 18, 35, 209

Hernfield, Rob 8, 225

Hope-Brown, Sinead 31-32

Hultgren, Mal 9, 76, 106, 173, 214

Hutson, Alexandria 35

I - J

Iverson, Amy J. 155

Jean, Ryan 115

Jennings, Amy 184, 222

Jerman, Candice 129

Johnson, Michael 239-241, 261-263

Jones, Christine 248

K

Kaplan, Kat   26-28

Kent, Saahah   59, 125, 219, 230, 238, 273

L

Lee, Laura   267

Lou, Claire   40-41

M

M.E.   265

Mackenzie, Jack   15

Mae, Julia   107-108

Matthews, Charlotte   30

McCarthy, Kirsty   8, 34, 42, 79, 127, 129, 174

McDonnell, Keriann   164

Murray, Jessica   226

N

Nappi, Eleonora   19-21, 50, 70, 100-101, 126, 131-132, 175, 176-179, 210-213, 220-221, 274-275

Natalie   66

Nielson, Tania   34, 38, 80-81, 93, 116, 128, 228, 260, 267

O

O'Rourke, Ashley   145

Oliver, Harry   258

P

Payne, Sammy   84

Potter, Jolene   188-204

Potter, Monique   36-37, 47-49, 71, 102-103, 123-124, 215, 218, 227, 254-255, 268-269

Purvis, Jennifer   3, 18, 74, 82, 138, 259, 266

Q - R

Quinney, Leanne 11-12

Reckless, Liliana Beth 33, 122, 185-186

Reyborn, Tiffany 3

Richard, Livia 16, 78, 92, 209, 272

Rodriguez, Yanelis E. 146-147

S

ScHarna 43

Scharples, Charlotte 229

Schulze, Shannon 95, 149-151

Simpson, Carly 4-5

Simpson, Krista 216, 244-246

Stampe, Karine 237

T

Taylor, Tee 29, 91, 130, 180, 205, 223, 243

The Catalyst 136-137

Trenaman, Michelle 118-119

V

Vanrell, Ann Font 256, 258

Vea Sommervold, Ida Emilee 266

W

Whitaker, Mary L. 120-121, 250-251

White, Cody 249

Wiliams, Star 25, 94

Wilson, Mel 51-52

Wood, Aimee 13-14

Wright, Carissa 85-90